# ABOUT THE AUTHORS

## MARYON STEWART

Maryon studied preventive dentistry and nutrition at the Royal Dental Hospital in London and worked as a counsellor with nutritional doctors in England for four years. She set up the PMT Advisory Service at the beginning of 1984 to bring nutritional help to all women sufferers of this under-acknowledged condition. Under her direction, the PMT Advisory Service provided help to thousands of women all over the world, a medical information service for doctors and other health workers, and a clinical trials unit. In February 1987 she launched the Women's Nutritional Advisory Service, which now provides broader help to women. Maryon has three children and is married to Dr Alan Stewart.

## SARAH TOOLEY

Sarah trained as a nurse in Sussex. After leaving the NHS in 1984 she joined the PMT Advisory Service shortly after its birth (now the WNAS). She gives nutritional advice to women in her WNAS clinics in London and Hove as well as postal advice to women on a national and international basis. For the past five years she has been senior nurse at the WNAS. Sarah has worked closely with Maryon and previously made major contributions to the menu and recipe sections of *The Vitality Diet* and *Beat PMT through Diet* books.

Also by Maryon Stewart:

*Beat PMT Through Diet*
*The Vitality Diet*

# BEAT PMT COOKBOOK

*Delicious recipes and weekly menus from the Women's Nutritional Advisory Service*

Maryon Stewart
with Sarah Tooley

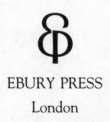

EBURY PRESS

London

*To Phoebe, Hester and Rebecca*
*– the young women of tomorrow.*

First published by Ebury Press
an imprint of the Random Century Group
Random Century House
20 Vauxhall Bridge Road
London SW1V 2SA

British Library Cataloguing in Publication Data
Stewart, Maryon
Beat PMT cookbook.
1. Women. Premenstrual syndrome. Therapy. Diet
I. Title II. Tooley, Sarah
618.1720654

ISBN 0–85223–926–2

Phototypeset in Goudy Old Style by Textype Typesetters, Cambridge
Printed and bound in Great Britain by Mackays of Chatham, Plc, Kent

# CONTENTS

## IMPORTANT NOTE FOR SUFFERERS

If you have symptoms which occur at other times of the month, apart from during your pre-menstrual time, you should have a medical check-up with your own doctor. If your symptoms are very severe it would be advisable to have your nutritional programme supervised by your own doctor or a trained counsellor. If you get confused or need extra advice, the Women's Nutritional Advisory Service is there to help you. All letters receive a personal reply: their address is on page 184.

## ACKNOWLEDGMENTS

We would like to thank Dr Guy Abraham and Dr Alan Stewart for their pioneering work in the field of nutrition and PMT, which has made our job so much easier.

Thanks are also due to Lavinia Trevor for her guidance, and to Rowena Webb and Amelia Thorpe at Ebury Press for their professionalism and enthusiasm.

This book would not have been possible without the wonderful feedback we have had over the years from our patients far and wide.

We are grateful to Jenny Tooley for her typing skills, Jane Booker for caring for the children whilst we worked, and Michele and Mike for their help. We would also like to acknowledge and thank the dedicated team of 'girls' at the Women's Nutritional Advisory Service for their hard teamwork and support over the years.

# INTRODUCTION

It is an established fact that dietary factors are closely related to our health. It is accepted that dietary changes can prevent heart disease, and play a major role in the control of diabetes and kidney disease. Experts now agree that the nutritional approach to Pre-Menstrual Syndrome, or PMT as it is more commonly known, is the best first-line treatment. In other words, by making dietary changes it is possible that you can alleviate your PMT symptoms to some degree.

What is not widely known, or appreciated, is just how one goes about making dietary changes, and what specific changes to the diet need to be made in order to overcome the different types of symptoms that women experience. For example, the dietary recommendations for overcoming breast tenderness would be somewhat different from the recommendations that would help abdominal bloating or irritability.

The Women's Nutritional Advisory Service has been giving dietary advice to women all over the world since 1984. The WNAS, formerly the PMT Advisory Service, has personally helped over thirty thousand women overcome their symptoms using the nutritional approach. From a study of two hundred WNAS patients, it was established that 96.5 per cent of the patients felt significantly better after the initial three months of following the recommendations. The WNAS programme is detailed in the successful companion to this book *Beat PMT Through Diet*.

This book concentrates on the different types of dietary changes that apply to the various types of symptoms. It is based on the extensive first-hand experience that we have gained from working with the women who over the years have come to us for help at the WNAS.

This special cookbook is designed to help you to help yourself. If this is your first encounter with the nutritional approach to PMT, you will need to read through the diet section and pick out the diet that is recommended for the majority of your symptoms. If you suffer with more than one category of symptoms you will need to combine several sets of recommendations initially. Read the book once through first, and then go back to the relevant sections to pick out the dietary recommendations most suitable for you.

If you have read *Beat PMT Through Diet*, or have in fact been on the WNAS programme, you will be able to use this book as a source of further ideas for meal planning. There are menus accompanying each section, and over one hundred recipes in all to choose from.

We wish you well over your symptoms, and hope you enjoy trying the recipes we have selected for you.

PART I

# THE PROBLEM

# 1

# PMT – A FORCE TO BE RECKONED WITH

PMT, or more correctly Pre-Menstrual Syndrome, is a collection of symptoms that occur before your period. These symptoms usually start between the time you ovulate – when the egg is released by the ovary in the middle of your cycle – and the time your period begins. The symptoms occur each month before a period, and classically disappear shortly after the onset of the period.

Whilst some fortunate women do not experience any PMT symptoms, a WNAS survey of women picked at random in the street indicated that some 73.6 per cent of women in Great Britain suffer to some degree. That translates into approximately 10 million women, some 7 million of whom are reckoned to experience moderate or severe pre-menstrual symptoms. So if it's any comfort, you are not suffering alone!

It is only now that we are beginning to realize the extent to which PMT symptoms affect the lives of sufferers. In November 1988, the WNAS conducted a survey on two hundred patients, all of whom had moderate to severe PMT symptoms. The survey discovered that relationships were commonly affected by symptoms – in fact, 96 per cent of the women surveyed felt that their home life or relationship with their family and friends was affected by their symptoms. Ninety-four per cent of the women felt depressed premenstrually, 75 per cent admitted to feeling violent and aggressive before their period, and 91 per cent felt that their productivity and efficiency at work decreased for an average of five days per month.

We discovered, very sadly, that of this group 53 per cent had contemplated suicide at least once pre-menstrually, and a staggering 11 per cent had actually attempted suicide at this time. It is quite clear from these statistics that PMT symptoms have a very significant effect on family members as well as on the sufferer herself.

We are often asked why it is that PMT seems to be more common nowadays than in years gone by. To that question there are indeed many answers. PMT has in fact existed for hundreds of years. We probably talk about it far more today, so it is recognized as being a common complaint. However, there are major factors that need to be considered when looking for the causes of PMT symptoms.

Firstly, you must appreciate that our nutritional state today is to some degree an inherited state, one that has been influenced by our physical experiences to date, plus a reflection of our lifestyle to some degree.

## THE PRODUCT OF PAST GENERATIONS

People often ask why it is that, although they eat well, they do not feel or look as well as someone they know who drinks, smokes and eats junk food. The fact is that although we can influence our nutritional condition by adjusting our diets now, we are the nutritional product of many generations. Our ancestors' bad habits or inadequate nutritional state can have a direct bearing on what 'material' we each have to start with. There is not a great deal we can do to influence this factor, but it does help to bear it in mind.

## THE PHYSICAL CHALLENGE

There is little doubt that physical experiences, especially those of a hormonal nature, take their toll on our bodies, unless of course we are one of the minority of educated individuals who know how to counteract the effects of pregnancy and breastfeeding, for example. We are not taught enough about nutritional requirements in general at school, let alone nutritional requirements for special situations. In fact we tend to know more about the needs of our cars than those of our bodies.

There are increased nutritional requirements during pregnancy and again during breastfeeding. If these are not adequately met, then the nutrients are passed from the mother's body to the infant. Over a period of time the mother then suffers lowered levels of certain key nutrients. When the body has borderline levels of important nutrients, or it in fact becomes deficient, it cannot function in an optimum fashion; conditions like PMT then occur even in women who may not previously have experienced them. Repeating this scenario in the second and possibly third pregnancy only serves to make the matter worse. Thus it is not uncommon to hear that PMT becomes worse after the second or third pregnancy.


## NUTRITIONAL STATE INFLUENCES HORMONE LEVELS

Research now shows us that nutritional factors can influence hormone levels in the body. To this day doctors fail to agree on the actual cause of PMT. Many feel that it is due to a hormone in-balance – probably low levels of the hormone progesterone. How-ever, some others think that it may be to do with the hormone oestrogen; whilst yet others consider that PMT is a disturbance of brain chemicals. Doctors often give hormone therapy in order to overcome the PMT symptoms, but what they are actually doing is masking the symptoms. For when the hormone treatment ceases, the symptoms return.

With the nutritional approach we are looking for the actual cause of the symptoms. Once we have found the cause we then address the problem and correct it by replacing the vitamins and minerals that are in short supply, so that the symptoms are eliminated on a permanent basis without having to resort to drugs at all, either in the short or long term.

This balance of hormones is affected by the ovaries, the liver and by normal bowel function.

Vitamin B and the type of diet we eat are also important.

Vitamin B appears to be necessary in the breakdown of oestrogen by the liver. Together with the minerals zinc and magnesium vitamin B also influences tissues, such as the lining of the womb, respond to oestrogen.

The balance of fibre and fat in the diet can affect the level of oestrogen in the blood.

Changing from an average western diet to a diet high in fibre and low in saturated (animal) fats can lower oestrogen levels. This may be desirable for women with PMT and especially for those with breast problems.

In this way changing and improving your diet can help to regulate hormone levels and thus control PMT symptoms in the long term.

## TWENTIETH-CENTURY LIFESTYLE

For many of us the twentieth century has brought a distinct change in lifestyle. We no longer have the extended family to fall back on, and we are often expected to go out to work as well as run a home and care for children. From time to time we may well experience stressful situations, like moving house, difficulties with children, financial or marital problems, or indeed just the stress of life in the fast lane.

Stress has an adverse effect on the body. It may even place increased nutritional demands on the body. Additionally, if we are overstretched and harassed we are far more likely to rely on pre-prepared processed food rather than indulging in home cooking, or we may indeed even eat sweet food in excess as a comfort. These types of foods contain less in the way of good nutrients, and in some cases even block the absorption of good nutrients from other foods.

It is also likely that when time is short, and we are overburdened, we have less time to exercise regularly. Exercise is very important. It has a proven beneficial effect – especially in helping to overcome symptoms of depression, anxiety and fatigue. Exercising is one of the few natural ways to speed up your metabolism, which is a very important consideration if you tend to put on weight. Regular exercise also is an excellent way to improve your general feeling of wellbeing.

# 2

# UPTIGHT, BLOATED AND DEPRESSED?

Pre-Menstrual Syndrome is a rather unusual condition as there are so many different sorts of symptoms that may be associated with it – it is thought that there are possibly in the region of 150. Most sufferers experience a few of the symptoms on a regular basis, and perhaps a few other symptoms some months, but not necessarily every month.

At WNAS we use a system of classifying symptoms which was devised by Dr Guy Abraham, a former professor of obstetrics and gynaecology from the University of California in Los Angeles. This classification works quite well, and helps us to some extent to select the type of diet and nutritional supplements that would be most suitable. There are four main groups of symptoms. Put a tick against the symptoms that you suffer on a regular basis:

## GROUP A (Anxiety)

| | Tick |
|---|---|
| Nervous tension | — |
| Mood swings | — |
| Irritability | — |
| Anxiety | — |

## GROUP H (Hydration)

Weight gain           ——
Swelling of extremities      ——
Breast tenderness        ——
Abdominal bloating       ——

## GROUP C (Cravings)

Headache             ——
Craving for sweets       ——
Increased appetite       ——
Heart pounding         ——
Fatigue              ——

## GROUP D (Depression)

Depression           ——
Forgetfulness          ——
Crying               ——
Confusion            ——
Insomnia             ——

It is possible that all of your symptoms fell into one group – but is unlikely. It is very common to suffer symptoms from more than one group, and indeed many women suffer symptoms from all four groups. Before deciding on the type of diet you should follow you will need to complete the following questionnaire. Your answers to the questions will give you the key to which dietary recommendations you should be following:

# SYMPTOM QUESTIONNAIRE

**1.** Are most of your symptoms mild? (Score one)          Score

*(Mild is defined as symptoms present that you are aware of, but they do not prevent you from carrying out all your usual activities.)*

**2.** Are most of your symptoms moderate? (Score three)

*(Moderate is defined as symptoms present that change the way you feel to the point where you occasionally cancel arrangements, and the family usually know your period is coming before you do.)*

**3.** Are many of your symptoms severe? (Score six)

*(Severe is defined as life-shattering symptoms. When they occur you are unable to carry on with your usual routine – in fact, you feel quite unable to cope until the symptoms have passed.)*

**Score three for each of the following questions:**

**4.** Would you describe yourself as Jekyll and Hyde (like two different people), one before your period and another after your period has begun?

**5.** Do you find it difficult to control your emotions when your symptoms are present?

**6.** Do you feel that your symptoms are spoiling your relationship with your partner or your children?

**7.** Do you feel that your symptoms affect your efficiency or productivity at work?

**8.** Do you find life generally difficult to cope with before your period arrives?

Total score          _____

## DID YOU SCORE THREE OR UNDER?

If you scored three or less you will almost certainly only need to follow the diet designed for mild sufferers. It seems that your PMT problems are under control, but you will probably benefit generally from the dietary changes. Refer to page 53 for your recommendations.

## DID YOU SCORE SIX OR UNDER?

You fall into the category of a moderate sufferer. You will need to make the specific dietary changes that are outlined on page 60. In addition you may be advised to take some of the recommended nutritional supplements, which you can read about on page 46.

## DID YOU SCORE SEVEN OR MORE?

You are obviously suffering severe symptoms. You will need to answer the next set of questions very carefully, and then follow the dietary recommendations beginning on page 68. You will need to take the recommended nutritional supplements for at least six months to help boost the nutritional levels in your body.

# FURTHER QUESTIONS FOR SEVERE SUFFERERS

1.   Do you suffer regularly with any two or more of the following symptoms pre-menstrually? (Score one for each)

Score

Abdominal bloating

Excessive wind

Constipation

Diarrhoea

Depression

Mouth ulcers

Fatigue

If you scored more than two in this section, you will need to follow the specific recommendations for a wheat-restricted diet on page 32.

**2.** Do you suffer any of the following symptoms? (Score one for each)

Score

Itchy bottom

Bloated abdomen

Cracking at the corners of your mouth

Depression

Excessive wind

Cystitis

Have you had more than two episodes of thrush in the last five years?

If you scored more than two in this section, or if you have had more than two episodes of thrush in the last five years, you will need to follow the recommendations for a yeast-restricted diet on page 34.

**3.** Would you describe mood swings and irritability as being two symptoms that you suffer especially severely? If the answer is yes, you will need to pay special attention to the extra recommendations on page 39.

**4.** Do you suffer severe breast tenderness for at least three to four days, practically every month, before your period begins? If your answer to this question is yes, you will need to pay particular attention to the extra recommendations on page 42.

**5.** (a) Does your desire to eat sweet foods increase pre-menstrually?
(b) Does your consumption of sweet foods or drinks at least double pre-menstrually?

If the answer to either of these questions is yes, you will need to follow the special recommendations on page 35 as well.

**6.** (a) Is your only pre-menstrual symptom depression? In other words, do you experience depression and not other symptoms before your period is due?

(b) Does your depression occur all through the month practically every day of your menstrual cycle (from the day your period
begins until your next period is due)?

If the answer to either of the above questions is yes, you will need to follow the advice given on page 40.

# PART II

# THE DIET

# 3

# A LITTLE KNOWLEDGE GOES A LONG WAY

For hundreds of years the knowledge that we have acquired about diet has been passed down from generation to generation. Different cultures obviously had different views on what the optimum diets were, but the information was at best intuitive, rather than scientifically based. Today we are very fortunate in that we have the scientific ability to determine what a good diet actually is. We can measure the harm that poor-quality foods bring about, and we can measure the value of good food to the body.

Before doing another weekly shop it is important to understand how the food and drink that you are about to consume might affect you. Obviously you will shop according to your taste and your pocket, and to some degree according to the traditions that have been set by your family. But there are certain groups of foods that should get a special mention right here at the outset as there clearly seems to be a relationship between them and adverse symptoms. These relationships are dealt with in greater detail in Chapter 4.

## ANIMAL FAT

It is widely recognized that our diet contains too much animal fat, which is often known as saturated fat. Animal fat is associated with heart disease, obesity and breast cancer. It also seems to aggravate many of the PMT symptoms. Animal fat should be replaced with polyunsaturated fat – cold-pressed oils such as sunflower or safflower, and spreads such as Vitaquel or Flora.

## FIBRE

In general our diets are too low in the right sort of fibre. The fibre we have been brainwashed to regard as healthful is bran. But we now know that bran blocks the absorption of several essential minerals, and aggravates many abdominal symptoms like bloating, wind, constipation and diarrhoea. You will be far better off increasing your consumption of salad, vegetables and fruit, all of which contain goodly amounts of vitamins and minerals. If bran is currently your solution to constipation, you can replace it with a daily dose of linseeds. These are available from the health food shop in the form of Linusit Gold. One to two tablespoons of linseeds with fruit and a little yogurt makes a delicious breakfast or snack and will more than adequately replace the laxative function of bran.

## SALT

We use between ten and twenty times more salt than our bodies actually require. Salt consumption is directly related to water retention in the body and to high blood pressure. If you are an addict, to start with you will need to use a replacement product like Lo Salt, but as soon as possible try to stop using salt altogether in your cooking or at the table, especially if you are prone to retain water pre-menstrually.

## SUGAR

In the UK alone we consume about 36 kg (80 lb) of sugar each per year. Apart from craving sweet food, we eat all sorts of food that contains hidden sugar. Sugar too promotes water retention in the body, and for this reason as well as many others is best avoided. It is a food that is empty of good nutrients, and in fact excessive consumption of sweet food may even impede the absorption of these nutrients.

## TEA, COFFEE AND COLA-BASED DRINKS

Tea, coffee and cola-based drinks contain high levels of caffeine and tannin. Both of these compounds are known to block the absorption of many essential nutrients. They are all addictive drinks which exacerbate symptoms of anxiety, nervous tension, insomnia and breast tenderness. Each cup of tea contains approximately 75 mg of caffeine and each cup of coffee about 90 mg. An intake in excess of 250 mg of caffeine per day can cause many adverse symptoms. We therefore recommend that tea and coffee should be reduced to a maximum of two or three cups per day, preferably a decaffeinated variety.

If you suffer anxiety, irritability, mood swings, nervous tension, insomnia or breast tenderness it is really advisable for you to give up these drinks altogether. If you are used to drinking several cups a day you may well experience headaches, irritability and even mild shakes as you attempt to eliminate them from your diet. These symptoms, if they occur, will pass within a week or two at the most – maybe even within a few days. On page 81 you will find a list of pleasant alternative drinks to try. Keep an open mind as you work your way through the list. You will be amazed at how quickly your tastes adapt once you have made the decision to make the changes.

## JUNK FOOD

Processed foods and TV dinners are promoted as a fast and convenient alternative to home cooking. It is easy to see how the glossy promotion of fast foods makes them attractive to many of us who have very busy lifestyles or who simply prefer the easy way out. Unfortunately, the processing of these meals greatly reduces the vitamin and mineral content of the basic ingredients. When eaten on a regular basis, these foods may even prevent good nutrients from other foods from being absorbed.

## MEAT

Although red meat was regarded by our ancestors as being one of the best – if not *the* best – type of food to consume, we now know that it should be consumed in moderation. The type of red meat available to us today is often too fatty, and may well have been contaminated with crop spray, antibiotics, even, possibly, growth hormones, all of which are undesirable to our bodies. Meat infected with BSE, better known as mad cow disease, is another current worry. You will probably feel a great deal better if you limit your intake of red meat to a maximum of three portions of organic or additive-free meat per week. Better still, eat free-range chicken and fish instead.

Additive-free meat is available from many butchers, and can sometimes be bought directly from a farm shop. Wild fish is preferable to farmed fish. Free-range eggs are a far better option than battery or other eggs which often contain antibiotics and could be contaminated with salmonella.

## ADDITIVES

Our bodies were not designed to cope with many of the chemical additives in the form of artificial colourings, stabilizers, flavour enhancers and preservatives that are now found in many of our foods. Whilst some are not harmful, the long-term effects of many of them on the human body are unknown. It is far better to avoid additives wherever possible.

## OTHER ENVIRONMENTAL FACTORS

The Ministry of Agriculture, Fisheries and Food admitted in a recent document that 99 per cent of all fruit and vegetables are treated at least once with some form of crop spray. There are many known environmental factors that can affect our food – anything from insecticides to nitrates in the soil or lead in petrol to airborne pollution. Apart from actively campaigning to lessen these harmful factors over the years, there is little we can do on a day-to-day basis other than learning how to choose the best food possible.

Organically grown fruit and vegetables are preferable to those that have been chemically sprayed. These are now available in most supermarkets. But nothing tastes better than home-grown produce – so if you have space in your garden or access to a plot of land, invest in a book on organic gardening (see page 180) and get to work. If you haven't the time to garden yourself, try to persuade a friend or relative to do the work in exchange for your supplying the materials. You can then share the produce.

## SOCIAL POISONS

Sadly, many of our social habits also affect our nutritional state. For example, alcohol blocks the absorption of most good nutrients, and should be avoided where possible. The maximum allowance of alcohol is three units per week, in other words three glasses of wine, or three measures of spirit, or three half pints of beer or lager. If you suffer particularly with breast tenderness, migraine or insomnia it would be worth cutting out alcohol altogether for at least an initial three-month period.

The social poisons also cover tobacco, drugs and even tea and coffee. It might amaze you to know that for every £1 spent on food in the UK, 76p was spent on alcohol and tobacco!

## DRINKING WATER

Disturbingly, it is now accepted that drinking water in many areas contains pollutants which are undesirable and often harmful to our bodies in the long term. The quality of the drinking water in many parts of the UK does not meet World Health Organization standards, particularly with regard to the high levels of lead and nitrates that are present. A slow accumulation of lead may affect child development and intelligence, and the nitrates are thought to increase the risk of cancer. It makes great sense to invest in an efficient water filter, which can be plumbed into the mains by your kitchen tap. A good water purifier will remove the vast majority of the harmful elements from the water.

## THE LAST STRAW

It is very disheartening to realize that even after going to all the trouble of growing your own vegetables and buying additive-free food, the cooking process destroys up to half the vitamins and mineral content of the food. It is just one of those facts that must be taken into account when planning balanced meals and menus. Grilling and steaming food causes less nutritional loss than frying, boiling and baking. It makes good sense to eat as much raw food as possible in order to get the full nutritional benefit. Plenty of salads, raw or lightly steamed vegetables and fruit will help to build up your vitamin and mineral intake.

## THE PAY-OFF

Whilst we admit that it does take time and effort to ring the changes, if you are sufficiently interested in your own health, and in the health and welfare of your family, you should have all the incentive you are likely to need. Some people like to start by making gradual changes; others prefer to make a clean sweep. Make the changes in the way that you feel you could best cope with and stick to in the long term. Changing long-standing habits is not an easy task, but it is not an impossible task either, especially when you have the vested interest of overcoming your symptoms as well as becoming more healthy generally.

# 4

# THE NUTRITIONAL
# PROGRAMME THAT
# CHANGES LIVES

When we set out in 1984 to help women overcome their PMT symptoms, we had little idea about the workability and effectiveness of the nutritional programme. We knew from published medical literature that specific nutritional supplements and dietary changes would help alleviate symptoms to some degree. It was not until we saw women completing their nutritional programme that we began to realize just how effective this method of treatment was.

As time went on we realized that we were transforming even the most desperate and suicidal PMT sufferers back into normal, balanced, happy human beings. Women who had previously described themselves as 'Jekyll and Hyde' were claiming that they felt stable all month and better than they could remember feeling since their youth. Husbands wrote to us gratefully claiming that they had 'got back the girl they married'. Many broken relationships 'mended', and very often found a new lease of life, once the woman was over her symptoms. Women, with reports verified by their husbands, claimed that their previously diminished or non-existent sex drive had risen to new improved levels.

Children stopped being afraid of their mothers, wondering whether they were about to lash out – although most of them spent many a nervous month watching carefully and waiting for mum to change back into an irrational monster. Women who had previously been afraid to work had successfully taken on responsible jobs outside the home. Even those who had previously suffered from agoraphobia for as long as ten years, as well as PMT, were now making regular solo outings to visit the hairdressers and the shops. Many women who had previously become dependent on tranquillizers or anti-depressants were managing to stop their medication, under the supervision of their doctors, without experiencing withdrawal symptoms.

The 'magic' continued as the years rolled on. In the first analysis of the nutritional programme, we found that 79 per cent of the women felt that their symptoms were completely or almost completely gone after three months on the nutritional programme. More recently, in a study of two hundred patients, we found that 96.5 per cent of the women who followed the recommendations felt significantly or completely better within three months.

The programme we use at the WNAS consists of five key elements:

1.  Specific dietary changes according to individual symptoms.
2.  Specialized nutritional supplements according to symptoms.
3.  Regular 'aerobic' exercise which includes anything from brisk walking, swimming, cycling and jogging to actual aerobic workouts.
4.  Lifestyle counselling to address day-to-day living and help to put life back on to an even keel where necessary.
5.  The WNAS helpline, which is there to give extra help and advice when necessary.

The programme is designed for moderate to severe patients who are not confident that they can help themselves. It is a four-month course of treatment designed not only to help the woman over her symptoms, but also to arm her with enough education on the subject of diet to carry her through life.

The programme operates from clinics and on a postal basis for those who are unable to get to a clinic. The postal service has been running successfully for many years and has helped women all over the world.

Women who suffer mild to moderate PMT can help themselves with diet, exercise and specific nutritional supplements (see page 46). The WNAS programme is described in some detail in the book *Beat PMT Through Diet*.

# SENSITIVITIES

Symptoms of PMT can be worsened by certain foods or other external factors, some of which have already been mentioned in passing in Chapter 3.

## COFFEE

Heart pounding, nervous tension, irritability, insomnia and diarrhoea.

## TEA

Heart pounding, nervous tension, irritability, insomnia and constipation.

## ALCOHOL

Headaches, rash, stomach upsets.

## MAKE-UP

Itching, dry flaking skin, soreness.

## PERFUME

Headaches, rashes.

## VARIOUS FOODS (see below)

Abdominal bloating, excessive wind, diarrhoea, constipation, weight gain and other symptoms.

For this reason, when certain symptoms are present it is best to avoid the suspect product or food all month until your PMT symptoms are under control.

## GRAINS

Among foods, certain grains can be particularly troublesome. A sensitivity to wheat, oats, barley, rye or corn can cause or aggravate the following symptoms: abdominal bloating, excessive wind, constipation, diarrhoea, depression, mouth ulcers and fatigue.

If you experience any of these symptoms exclude whole wheat and whole wheat products from your diet initially. If your symptoms persist, you will need to exclude the other grains too for a period of four weeks. Since corn and rice are the two grains with which women find the least problems, unless you feel they upset you it is fine to include them in your diet initially.

### What to avoid

**Wheat**   Bread, pasta, cakes, biscuits, pastry, pies, buns, breakfast cereals and sausages.

**Oats**   Porridge, oat cookies and oat flakes.

**Rye**   Rye bread (which also contains wheat) and Ryvita.

**Barley**   Found in packet/tinned soups and stews, and barley beverages.

**Corn**   Corn on the cob, corn starch, cornflour, corn (maize) oil and popcorn.

The rule is to read labels in the supermarket, as flour, edible starch and so on are added to many processed foods.

### Assessing for a sensitivity

If you have cut any grains from your diet because you feel you may be allergic to them, avoid whole wheat for six to eight weeks before attempting to reintroduce it; then bring back the grains one at a time. This should be done after your period or in the symptom-free phase of your cycle, so that any possible reaction will not be confused with PMT. Eat your first reintroduced grain at least once or twice a day for five days. If you do not experience any reaction after five days, stop eating that grain and try another one. This introducing phase can take two months or more, depending on the length of your cycle and symptoms.

If you experience a reaction to a particular grain it does not mean that you will never be able to eat this food again – simply that your body is reacting at present. Once your nutritional state has improved, you should find that your body is better able to tolerate this food. It is important to remember, however, that you can be more sensitive when pre-menstrual; therefore there may be some foods that you need to avoid or cut down on at this time of the month until your PMT symptoms have reduced sufficiently.

### What to eat instead

A small amount of white bread or pasta

Potatoes and potato flour

Brown rice and rice flour

Rice cakes

Buckwheat and buckwheat flour

You can still eat a small amount of white flour daily. This is not because white flour is better for you, but because it has been refined and most of the whole grain (and goodness) has been removed. It is the whole wheat that seems to cause a sensitivity.

Alternative flours are available from health food shops and can be used in cooking:

Soya flour

Buckwheat flour

Rice flour

Potato flour

Often trial and error are necessary to obtain the correct texture for cooking with these flours. We recommend them if you have established that you have a sensitivity to a particular grain, or in the short term whilst you are avoiding wheat and possibly oats, barley and rye.

Larkhall Laboratories supply Trufree Flours, available from some chemists, which give particularly good results in baking. There is a very good cookery book called The Bumper Bake Book, which gives recipes for using these flours with good results (see page 180).

## Nutritional values

You should not lose any nutrients from avoiding these grains for the specified time, as there are many other foods that also supply nutrients. For example:

|  | Wholemeal bread | Broccoli tops | Soya flour |
|---|---|---|---|
|  | mg per 100g | | |
| Fibre | 8.5 | 4.1 | 14.3 |
| Calcium | 23 | 76 | 240 |
| Vitamin B6 | 0.14 | 0.13 | 0.68 |

Following the replacement diet plan on page 33 will help you to ensure a well-balanced diet.

The recipes in the recipe section are coded (W) for wholewheat-free and (G) for grain-free. You may find that you can use white flour in some of the recipes if you are not avoiding it.

## YEAST

A sensitivity to or excess of yeast can cause these symptoms: itchy bottom, bloated abdomen, cracking at the corners of the mouth, depression, excessive wind, cystitis and thrush.

Yeast is part of the normal make-up of the gut, and is balanced with bacteria to help perform the normal functions of our intestinal tract. Sometimes a yeast overgrowth can occur, causing toxins which can produce mental and physical symptoms. PMT symptoms such as confusion, fatigue, depression, poor memory and a general lethargy and unwell feeling can all be caused or aggravated by a yeast overgrowth. Long illnesses and/or repeated use of antibiotics can also cause the yeast bug to overgrow.

### What to avoid

**Sugar**   Sugary foods like cakes, biscuits and honey.

**Bread**   Bread, buns and any foods that have had yeast added to them.

| | |
|---|---|
| **Alcohol** | Most alcoholic drinks, especially beer, depend on yeast to produce the alcohol. |
| **Juices** | Citrus fruit juices – only freshly squeezed juice is yeast-free. You can, however, use the small cartons as long as the whole carton is consumed in one sitting. This is because once a large carton is opened yeast begins to form. |
| **Malt** | Malted cereals and drinks. |
| **Pickles** | Any pickles, sauerkraut, olives, chillies, vinegar and condiments containing vinegar. |
| **Cheese** | Blue cheeses and Brie. |
| **Fungi** | Mushrooms. |
| **Fruits** | All dried fruits and over-ripe soft fruits. |
| **Extracts** | Marmite and stock cubes. |

All fermented foods, leftover and stale foods also contain high amounts of yeast. It is very difficult to avoid yeast altogether as it is everywhere around us, but avoiding the above foods until the symptoms subside will help your body to correct its yeast balance. If you feel that your yeast problem is persistent you should consult your GP for oral medication to help.

As live natural yogurt contains bacteria which help to balance the yeast, it may be helpful to eat it two or three times per week.

Vegetable stock used in recipes should be made from the water vegetables have been cooked in which can then be frozen.

To help you follow a low-yeast diet, the menus and recipes in later chapters are coded with a (Y) to indicate that they are suitable for a low-yeast diet.

## SUGAR CRAVINGS

Craving for sweet food can be more than just a passing fancy. Very often people get addicted to sweet food, and the problem becomes worse pre-menstrually. It is not uncommon for severe sufferers to consume several chocolate bars per day or even a whole packet of biscuits at one sitting. The body needs sugar in the form of glucose in order for the brain to function and the cells to generate energy. Wholesome food is converted into glucose by the body.

Regular intakes of good food keep the blood sugar levels constant, which in turn keeps cravings for sweet food at bay. But regular 'injections' of refined sweet foods, like cakes, biscuits, sweets, chocolates and the non-diet variety of fizzy drinks, cause the blood sugar levels to rise rapidly and subsequently dip, which then creates a demand for more sweet food.

As refined sweet food is metabolized quickly, it only produces an initial spurt of energy. The sharp lowering of blood sugar is what induces symptoms of hunger, cravings and fatigue. Refined sweet foods are high in calories, but relatively empty of nutrients. They also impede the absorption of nutrients from the good food you may also be eating.

Sweet cravings can be overcome permanently, within a few months. However, it is not an easy task and therefore needs approaching in a very controlled manner. But don't be discouraged – the WNAS has had tremendous success with overcoming sweet cravings.

## EFFECTS OF SUGAR

PMT C – headaches, cravings for sweets, increased appetite, heart pounding, fatigue, and dizziness or fainting. All these symptoms can be associated with poor blood sugar control. Mood swings and irritability are also common reactions.

It is important therefore to maintain good blood sugar control without using refined sugars. This does not mean that you can never eat a piece of chocolate cake again – these things are fine in small quantities once your symptoms have reduced and are under control.

### The mineral chromium

It has been found that a trace mineral called chromium can play an important role in blood sugar metabolism. Ensure that you are eating a diet rich in chromium by including some of the following foods in your diet: apples, bananas, green peppers, parsnips, potatoes, spinach, eggs, calves' liver, chicken, scallops, shrimps and black pepper.

### Dietary supplements can help

The WNAS has researched and formulated a special supplement called Sugar Factor, which is designed to normalize blood sugar levels. It contains optimum amounts of chromium and magnesium, both of which have been shown to help sugar cravings. In our experience it is ideal to take a supplement like Sugar Factor for about four months. It acts as a 'nutritional prop', which seems to be needed initially in order to control the blood sugar levels whilst establishing new eating patterns. More information on this supplement is given on page 48.

### How to maintain blood sugar levels

Eat small regular snacks and meals. Example:

| | |
|---|---|
| 7.30 am | breakfast |
| 10.30 am | mid-morning snack |
| 1.30 pm | lunch |
| 4.30 pm | mid-afternoon snack |
| 7.30 pm | dinner |
| 10 pm | light snack |

For some people this may strike a chord of horror with weight gain fears. This need not be so, and in fact we usually find that women lose weight on this kind of nutritional programme. Do not forget, also, that you are cutting out the high calories in sugary foods, and replacing these with more nutritious foods.

### Alternative snacks

Before unwrapping the next bar of chocolate stop and think – do you really want the symptoms of headache and fatigue that are likely to follow a few hours later, not to mention the weight gain and spotty skin that may develop? Try to choose from the following instead:

1. Rice cakes, either on their own or with a savoury or sweet topping such as mashed sardines or sliced bananas.

2. Rice salad, which can be cooked and made whilst you are cooking the evening meal and taken to work or kept in the

fridge for use the next day. A couple of tablespoons would provide a good snack. Chop nuts, peppers, fruit, celery or any salad vegetable into it to make it more interesting.

3.  Potato salad – again add chives, spring onions or chopped crisp Chinese leaves to make it more appetizing.

4.  Unsalted nuts or seeds – one or two tablespoons should satisfy your hunger, and they are also highly nutritious.

5.  Fresh fruit, particularly bananas, can satisfy your hunger.

6.  Low-sugar or sugar-free fruit and nut bars.

7.  Ryvita with a topping (if you are not avoiding grains). These do contain salt, so should be avoided two weeks pre-menstrually.

8.  Low-fat natural or live yogurt with added seeds or fruit. If you are following a low dairy diet remember that this comes out of your dairy allowance.

9.  Raw carrots or celery are nice and crispy to nibble on.

10. Goat's yogurt, provided you keep within your dairy allowance.

### What to avoid

Cakes, biscuits, sweet puddings, jams, jelly, ice cream, sweets, chocolate, and any packet foods such as breakfast cereals with sugar high on the ingredient list.

### What to use instead

**Sweeteners in drinks** are not ideal. Try to dispense with your sweet tooth gradually by slowly reducing the amount of sugar added to your drinks.

**Jams:** sugar-free jams are available from health food shops.

**Desserts:** you will find that many of the dessert recipes in this book are in fact made without sugar, and fresh fruit salads make a naturally sweet alternative.

**Drinks:** adding hot or cold water or carbonated water to fresh fruit juice makes a refreshing drink in place of sugary fizzy drinks.

**Snacks:** see above for alternatives to the tea-break chocolate or biscuit.

# MOOD SWINGS AND IRRITABILITY

These are problems that anyone can suffer from, perhaps when under stress, but it is the degree of suffering and frequency that make them more of a problem for PMT sufferers.

Many women find that their tolerance level is greatly reduced pre-menstrually and they frequently find themselves screaming, shouting or striking out at their husband, children or loved one for little or no reason. Sometimes an innocent comment or clumsy child can cause a severe reaction; had the same thing occurred at any other time of the month the incident would probably have gone unnoticed.

Mood swings and irritability are not just emotions that one can always control if 'one pulls oneself together'; they can often be caused by dietary factors and social poisons, especially pre-menstrually when your body is more susceptible. By simply reducing or, in a severe sufferer's case, avoiding completely the foods that may aggravate the feeling, the symptoms may greatly reduce or be eradicated altogether.

### What to avoid

**Tea**  Impedes the absorption of important nutrients, particularly iron, which is important to menstruating women. This can aggravate heart pounding, irritability, insomnia, constipation and tremors.

**Coffee**  Again, it impedes absorption of important nutrients and can also cause heart pounding, irritability, insomnia, diarrhoea and tremors.

**Sugar**  Sugary foods can affect your blood sugar levels, causing swings from high to low. It seems that pre-menstrually some women experience typical symptoms of hypoglycaemia (low blood sugar), which include mood swings and irritability, fatigue and depression.

**Alcohol**  As we all know, alcohol can affect our emotional state, making us perhaps very happy but in some circumstances hyper-sensitive, irritable and moody.

**Smoking**  Interferes with digestion, reduces vitamin C levels and causes irritability.

Try to keep all the above to a minimum, as they will only be tolerated in small amounts initially. If you have been a long-term smoker, it is probably better to get your new diet well and truly established and get your symptoms stabilized to some degree before attempting to cut down or give up smoking. The purpose of this approach is to avoid additional withdrawal symptoms occurring whilst you still have severe PMT symptoms.

### What to use instead

**Tea**　　There are many substitutes to suit all tastes – herby, fruity, flowery or simply decaffeinated.

**Coffee**　Decaffeinated coffee can be used as a substitute, but kept to a maximum of two cups per day. There are other chemicals in decaffeinated coffee besides caffeine, and these too can aggravate PMT symptoms.

**Sugar**　Substitutes are not always ideal, especially as you need to train your palate to accept less sugary-tasting foods. Try to cut down generally on sugar in drinks and foods and snacks containing sugar.

**Alcohol**　Social situations can make avoiding alcohol difficult. However, you should try to stick to mineral waters, fruit juices and alcohol-free wine or beer for now. You do have an alcohol allowance of three units per week if you are not a severe sufferer, but it should be avoided completely pre-menstrually.

There is an extensive list of alternatives on page 80.

# DEPRESSION AND CHRONIC (NON-CYCLIC) SYMPTOMS

If you feel that you experience severe depression pre-menstrually and this is your only real symptom, you should see your GP for advice and support.

Any menstruating woman or woman with ovaries is still producing hormones and is susceptible to PMT symptoms. This does not, however, mean that this is the sole cause of all her problems. We have often found that women with chronic complaints such as depression, fatigue, headaches/migraines, arthritis and even back-ache can find that their symptoms are worsened pre-menstrually.

If any of your symptoms do not appear to have a pattern or persist throughout the month it is important that you seek correct medical advice from your GP. There may be another cause which needs treatment.

## MIGRAINE AND HEADACHES

These can be particularly destructive, especially if they last for days. Some women have to retire to a darkened room, totally away from the family and work commitments.

Whether these are a chronic problem or cyclic, certain dietary changes can help. Severe blood sugar swings can trigger a headache/migraine. See advice on page 35.

### What to avoid

**Fruit**      Oranges have been known to be a cause; the fruit and juice should be avoided.

**Cheese**     Hard yellow cheeses especially.

**Yeast**      See the details of yeast foods to be avoided on page 34.

**Sugar**      This can start a headache by causing large blood sugar swings.

**Chocolate**  Not only will the sugar content cause headaches, but it also contains caffeine, another aggravating factor.

**Stress**     Not everyone can avoid stress in their lives, but it is important to try to recognize when you are under extra stress. You can then ensure you take better care of yourself, including relaxation techniques (see exercise on page 86).

**Fluids**     We know that the hangovers from excess alcohol can be caused by dehydration. When we lead busy lives it can be easy to forget to drink enough. Try to drink plenty of mineral water; ideally consume 2½ to 3 pints of fluid daily.

# BREAST PAIN AND TENDERNESS

If you have painful or lumpy breasts cyclically or all month you should see your GP for a check. All women should really check their own breasts monthly, whilst in the bath or lying in bed. Your local Family Planning Centre or GP's surgery will be able to supply you with a leaflet on how this should be done.

Severe breast tenderness can be a very distressing symptom for PMT sufferers. Even walking downstairs or giving the children a cuddle can cause pain. Different-size bras are often needed pre-menstrually due to the size increase and tenderness. Dietary factors again influence these symptoms and a change of diet can reduce them in two to three months.

### What to avoid

| | |
|---|---|
| **Smoking** | Simply stopping smoking can alleviate breast symptoms. |
| **Tea** | The chemicals in tea seem to aggravate the breast tissue. |
| **Coffee** | Again, chemicals can cause breast tenderness. |
| **Dairy** | Avoid a high dairy intake, as these foods can be high in saturated fats which can aggravate many breast conditions. |
| **Salt** | Salt added to cooking or at the table can aggravate fluid retention, which would worsen breast symptoms. |
| **Salty foods** | Salt is present in many foods, especially processed convenience foods: soups, ham, bacon, tinned fish in brine, crisps and even cheese. It is necessary to avoid as many of these foods as possible at present. You should particularly aim to avoid them in the two weeks before your period. |
| **Sugary foods** | These can cause hormonal changes, which in turn can affect the fluid balance in your body. |
| **Alcohol** | As alcohol has a chemical-like action on your body it will also affect breast tissue. Additionally it blocks the absorption of good nutrients. |

**Fatty foods**    Saturated fats should be kept down; they are con-
tained in foods such as red meat, mince, sausages,
hard margarines, lard, dripping suet, palm and
coconut oil and foods containing them. Always
remove the skin or fat from any meat, preferably
before cooking.

### What to eat instead

As well as following the general dietary recommendations for mild,
moderate or severe sufferers, essential fatty acids such as fish oils are
important in helping reduce breast symptoms. Oily fish are particularly important; try to have at least two to three portions per week
of fish such as herrings, mackerel, pilchards, salmon, sardines, sprats
and whitebait.

### Supplements

Evening Primrose Oil (Efamol) and natural vitamin E are of proven
benefit in easing breast tenderness. (See supplement recommendations on page 47.)

# PERIOD PAIN

This can be an added torment to PMT sufferers, but we have had
very good success in helping women overcome this problem. Diet,
exercise and supplements all play an important role. See page 179
for details of two very helpful books, *Coping with Periods* and *Pain-
free Periods*.

### Diet

Follow your PMT diet recommendations, which have been shown
also to help period pain sufferers.

### Exercise

This can improve blood supply. Gentle massage and heat to the
pelvic area, such as a warm hot water bottle, also improve circulation and can therefore reduce cramping.

### Smoking

This can worsen period pain and should be avoided, especially when experiencing the pain.

### Supplement

Optivite or the PMT supplement, and the diet recommendations have proven to be very helpful; sometimes an extra supplement of magnesium is also necessary. (See supplement recommendations on page 48.)

### Constipation

Many PMT sufferers find that they become constipated pre-menstrually; this can worsen the period pain and should therefore be avoided. Your diet programme should offer plenty of fresh vegetables, fruit and fibre; an adequate fluid supply and the use of linseeds are also important. Exercise again will help constipation.

## IRON-RICH DIET

## ANAEMIA

This is a condition that most women will have heard of – it simply means low iron. As women lose iron with their monthly menstruation, it is important to ensure that the body has an adequate supply. Heavy and long periods can both cause anaemia. You are likely to be particular susceptible if your diet is lacking in iron-rich foods or you are consuming substances that block the uptake of iron.

### Symptoms

Fatigue, sore tongue, and cracking at the corners of the mouth.

### What to do

If you do suffer from heavy and/or long periods you should seek your GP's advice. He may wish to give you an iron test, and if necessary prescribe a course of iron and investigate the possible causes of these problems.

Vegetarians and vegans can be particularly susceptible to anaemia due to the lack of red meat in their diets. There are, of course, diet-conscious and not so diet-conscious vegetarians (see page 77). Below is a list of foods that contain iron. Include a variety of these in your diet (avoiding for now those that are not permitted in your diet recommendations).

| | | |
|---|---|---|
| wheat bran | mussels | parsley |
| beef | scallops | spring greens |
| lamb | almonds | leeks |
| liver | brazil nuts | apricots |
| Bovril | coconut | bananas |
| egg yolk | haricot beans | blackberries |
| sardines | mung beans | dried figs |
| mackerel | kidney beans | raisins |
| crab | avocados | prunes |
| cockles | lentils | |

Vitamin C in your diet will increase your absorption of iron. It would therefore be preferable to eat some fruit such as an orange after your meal, or to have a glass of orange juice with your meal.

### What to avoid

**Tea**   Tea, if taken with a meal, blocks the absorption of two-thirds of the iron you would have absorbed from the vegetables in your meal. By drinking orange juice with your meal you will increase your iron absorption.

**Bran**   This will again block iron absorption, and is therefore best kept fairly low if you do have a persistent iron problem.

# 5

# SUPPLEMENTING THE DIET

If you have moderate to severe PMT symptoms you may well need to take some nutritional supplements, at least in the short term. Having said that, at the Women's Nutritional Advisory Service we do not advise people to take random supplements – in other words, a bit of this and a bit of that. The result of uneducated purchasing in the health food shop may leave you in an even more physically unbalanced and mentally confused situation. It is definitely not recommended.

There are a number of supplements that have been scientifically tried and tested over the years – we only recommend those that have been through properly conducted clinical trials. There are some which are best for general symptoms, and others which have more specialist uses. For example, the multi-vitamin and mineral preparations like Optivite, and PMT in Australia, New Zealand and Singapore, are good for general symptoms. Natural vitamin E is particularly good for breast symptoms, as is Evening Primrose Oil (Efamol), which is also effective in overcoming skin conditions. Extra vitamin C is advisable daily if you are a smoker. The supplement Sugar Factor may be useful if you experience pre-menstrual sugar cravings.

The information on the following pages will give you some idea of the strengths of key supplements in treating certain symptoms, and the dosages required.

## OPTIVITE

A multi-mineral and multi-vitamin formulation which is the most clinically tried and tested vitamin and mineral supplement in the world for PMT symptoms. It was formulated by Dr Guy Abraham, a former professor of obstetrics and gynaecology in California. It has been available for some ten years, and has helped many thousands of women.

### Daily dosage

Two to six tablets per day. If you have severe symptoms you will need to take four tablets per day, from the first day of your period until the middle of your cycle, when you increase to six tablets per day until your period arrives. For moderate sufferers the dosage would be lower – two to four tablets per day. Mild sufferers need only take one or two tablets per day.

### Availability

In the UK Optivite is available in Boots, other chemists and health food shops. For availability in other countries see page 186.

## EVENING PRIMROSE OIL (EFAMOL)

Evening Primrose oil has been the subject of a great deal of research. It has been shown to be extremely effective for the treatment of breast symptoms and skin conditions like eczema.

### Daily dosage

Between four and eight capsules per day.

### Availability

Evening Primrose oil is available in the UK in all chemist's and health food shops. It is also available in many other countries around the world (see page 186).

## NATURAL VITAMIN E

Natural vitamin E has also been the subject of medical research. It is of proven benefit in the treatment of skin conditions and breast tenderness.

### Daily dosage

The recommended daily dosage is 400 iu's (international units) per day.

## SUGAR FACTOR

This is a special combination of vitamins and minerals that have been put together to help overcome cravings for sweet food. The formulation is based on the research of the WNAS. It contains high levels of the mineral chromium, which has been shown to help normalize blood sugar levels.

### Daily dosage

One to two tablets per day, depending on severity of symptoms.

### Availability

Sugar Factor is available from Nature's Best (for details see page 185).

## MAGNESIUM

We have found this to be very helpful in dealing with period cramps. Magnesium is important to the muscles and can help reduce the cramps experienced at the time of the period.

### Daily dose

Magnesium amino-acid chelate, 125 mg, two to three daily every day of your cycle.

### Availability

Nature's Best and most chemist's or health food shops.

# 6

# A SIX-MONTH INVESTMENT

## THE SHORT TERM

Once you have selected the type of diet to follow, you need to stick to it as closely as possible for the first three months. If your symptoms are mild, you may not need to take nutritional supplements, as long as you keep to the diet. If, however, your symptoms are moderate to severe, you will undoubtedly need to take nutritional supplements for the first six months at least. Details of specific recommended supplements are in Chapter 5. Select your supplements and follow the recommendations carefully.

Exercise is of proven benefit, particularly for women suffering anxiety, irritability, insomnia and depression. Choose the exercises you enjoy, and work out a weekly routine for yourself. You need to exercise at least three or four times per week for at least forty minutes each time.

You might find it useful to chart your symptoms on a daily basis. It is handy to have records to refer to, rather than relying on your memory.

## THE MEDIUM TERM

After about three to four months your symptoms should be more or less under control. Once you have reached the point where you feel significantly better, you can start to adjust your diet and reduce the nutritional supplements gradually.

If you have been following a wheat-free or yeast-free diet, you can begin to reintroduce the foods you have been avoiding, one by one. Allow five to seven days between introducing new foods, so that any reactions you may have will be clearly attributable to a specific food. If you have been avoiding all grains, select one type of grain to try – wheat, for example. Include it in your diet for several days. If you do not experience any adverse reactions, wait a few days and then introduce the next grain.

If, whilst you are adding wheat to your diet, you experience 'old symptoms' again, be they fatigue, abdominal bloating, constipation, headaches or whatever, stop the wheat immediately and put it on your 'black list'. Return to your basic diet and wait a few days before trying the next type of grain, in order to avoid confusion.

Once you have experimented with the different types of food you had previously been avoiding, and have put together the diet that seems to suit your body, continue with it for another three months. Keep taking the nutritional supplements each day of your cycle, and continue with your exercise programme.

## SURVIVING SYMPTOM-FREE IN THE LONG TERM

Any diet and exercise programme, even when you are feeling well, only works if you happen to like the diet and the exercises you are following. If you are not keen on either the type of diet or the exercises, it is fairly obvious that you will not have the inclination to stick to the regime in the long term. Hopefully you will be happy with your new diet and exercise regime.

In our experience, women's tastes change so much during the first few months that they have little desire to return to their previous way of eating – or drinking, for that matter. It should be said, however, that we do not expect you to turn into a 'nutritional saint' forever. Once you have the certainty about what your body likes and dislikes on a regular basis, it is perfectly acceptable for you to 'cheat' when on holiday, on a special occasion or at a dinner party. If you do experience symptoms again after one of these episodes, then all you need to do is go back on the basic diet for a week or two, until you feel completely well again. After a while you will get to know your own body and what it requires of you.

Continue with your exercise routine as regularly as you possibly can. You will find that you feel so much better. If you need further information, consult the book *Beat PMT Through Diet*, and if you need further help and guidance you can contact us at the WNAS.

# LONG-TERM MANAGEMENT

Ideally, in the long term, it is preferable to manage with diet alone. However, you may feel that you would like to go on taking your supplements, perhaps on a reduced dosage, to safeguard against the return of symptoms and as an 'insurance policy' to maintain a good balance of health generally.

On long-term follow-up on WNAS patients we discovered that former PMT sufferers prefer to maintain their supplements in one of three ways:

**1.** To continue to take a reduced dosage of supplements every day of their menstrual cycle as an insurance.

**2.** To take supplements only on those days before the period when they would normally have had symptoms.

**3.** To take supplements only when under stress, or when travelling away from home and their normal diet.

It is really up to you to decide which long-term option you feel happiest with. You might like to start with Option 1 and work your way through to Option 3 over a few years. It is certainly felt that moderate daily dietary supplementation may well be a good idea in the long term, in view of the fact that so many nutrients are lost to the environment or in the process of cooking.

The following three chapters include sample menus for different degrees of symptoms. They need not be followed exactly on a daily basis, but will give you an idea of the range and types of foods you should be eating. Time and finances will play a part in your meal planning. You can adjust these examples to suit your requirements, as long as you keep within the guidelines of your particular diet recommendations. You will notice that some dishes are marked with an asterisk. This simply means that there is a recipe for the dish in the recipe section.

If you select a restricted diet to follow, you will need to look out for the specialized recipes. For example grain-free recipes will be marked with a G, low yeast recipes will be marked with a Y, and wholewheat-free recipes will be marked with a W. Vegetarian recipes can be found on page 78.

Write down your personal recommendations as you select them so you have them at hand for your reference. Before selecting a dish, check the list of ingredients in the recipe section to make sure that none of them is forbidden for you.

# 7

# RECOMMENDATIONS AND MENUS FOR MILD SUFFERERS

## TEA

Reduce intake of tea to a maximum of three weak cups per day.

## COFFEE

Only one cup of standard coffee and a maximum of three cups of decaffeinated coffee per day.

## ALCOHOL

Keep this to a maximum of three to four drinks per week, but avoid for one week before your period.

## RED MEAT

Keep to a maximum of three to four portions per week.

## DAIRY

Keep your dairy consumption down to a maximum of ½ pint per day (or equivalent – see page 82).

## SALT

Avoid adding salt at the table, and try to use salt substitute in cooking instead.

## VEGETABLES

Increase your consumption of greens and other fresh vegetables to at least once daily. Buy organic vegetables, or use home-grown where possible.

## WHOLEFOODS

Try to ensure that your diet contains plenty of wholefoods – unprocessed grains in the form of wholemeal bread, oats, rye and so on. Use fresh foods as opposed to frozen where possible (fresh fish instead of frozen fish fingers, for example). Good-quality natural vegetable oils should also be used in cooking, and vegetable margarines instead of too much butter.

## SUGAR

Keep sugar consumption low in the form of sugar added to drinks: try to reduce this gradually. Where sugary foods are concerned, let yourself have an occasional treat but not in the week before your period. Soft drinks also have a high sugar content, so reduce your consumption of these to two to three per week; again be careful in the week before your period, because of blood sugar swings (see page 35).

For help with keeping to this regime, see Chapter 10.

## SAMPLE MENUS

There are two weeks' worth of sample menus. If required, please use snacks of your choice from the snack list on page 37. For dessert have fresh fruit or select a suitable sweet from the section on page 165. The starred items will be found in the recipe section.

## DAY 1

Breakfast  Dried fruit compote*

Lunch  Jacket potato
Low sugar and salt baked beans

Dinner  Roast chicken with orange and herb sauce*
Chinese leave
Courgettes
Roast potatoes

## DAY 2

Breakfast  ½ grapefruit sprinkled with nuts
1 slice wholemeal toast with sugar-free jam

Lunch  Cottage cheese and salad sandwich made with
wholemeal bread

Dinner  Grilled turkey breast
Bean and sweetcorn salad*
Lettuce
Spicy lentil dressing*

## DAY 3

Breakfast  2 boiled eggs with 1 slice wholemeal toast
Live yogurt

Lunch  Grilled fillet of plaice
Grilled tomatoes
Broccoli
Mashed potatoes

Dinner  Spiced liver*
Brown rice

## DAY 4

Breakfast  Cornflakes
Apple juice
1 chopped apple

Lunch  Tuna jacket*
Green salad*

Dinner  Piquant pork chops*
Broccoli
Carrots
Boiled potatoes

## DAY 5

Breakfast  Poached egg on wholemeal toast

Lunch  Salmon potato cakes*
Beansprout salad*

Dinner  Grilled chicken with mustard sauce*
Spinach
Cauliflower
Brown rice

## DAY 6

Breakfast  Fresh fruit salad*
Yogurt

Lunch  Bean and carrot soup*
French bread

Dinner  Fish moussaka*
Green salad*

## DAY 7

Breakfast  Grilled mushrooms on wholemeal toast

Lunch  Grilled plaice
Peas
Grilled tomatoes
Sauté potatoes

Dinner  Steak with mixed herbs*
Spinach salad*
Jacket potato

## DAY 1

Breakfast  Fresh fruit salad*
Live yogurt

Lunch  Chilled tomato soup*
Wholemeal toast

Dinner  Herb-baked gammon*
Spinach
Sweetcorn
Roast potatoes

## DAY 2

Breakfast  Porridge made with water
1 chopped banana
1 tablespoon seeds or ground nuts

Lunch  Cold chicken breast
Waldorf salad*
Cold brown rice

Dinner  Plaice with yogurt and nuts*
Carrots
Red cabbage
Boiled potatoes

## DAY 3

Breakfast  Rice Krispies
1 chopped apple
Skimmed milk

Lunch  Tuna and salad sandwich made with wholemeal bread

Dinner  Lamb chops with rosemary*
Cabbage
Grilled tomatoes
Jacket potato

## DAY 4

Breakfast  Scrambled egg on wholemeal toast

Lunch  Cold turkey
Green salad*
Brown rice

Dinner  Fisherman's pie*
Peas
Sweetcorn

## DAY 5

Breakfast  Wholemeal toast
Sugar-free jam

Lunch  Jacket potato
2 oz grated cheese
Coleslaw salad*

Dinner  Grilled chicken with tomato sauce*
Red cabbage
French beans
Boiled potatoes

## DAY 6

Breakfast    Oats with skimmed milk
Chopped fresh fruit
1 tablespoon nuts

Lunch    Leek and potato soup*
French bread

Dinner    Mackerel with lemon stuffing*
Spinach
Carrots
Boiled potatoes

## DAY 7

Breakfast    2 boiled eggs
1 slice wholemeal bread

Lunch    Steamed cod's roe
Minty cabbage salad*
Potato salad*

Dinner    Beef and bean casserole*
Brown rice

# 8

# RECOMMENDATIONS AND MENUS FOR MODERATE SUFFERERS

### TEA

Only one or two weak cups per day.

### COFFEE

Avoid standard coffee, but up to two cups of decaffeinated per day.

### ALCOHOL

A maximum of one to two drinks per week, but avoid altogether for two weeks pre-menstrually.

### SMOKING

Try to stop smoking altogether.

### DAIRY

Keep consumption down to ½ pint total dairy allowance per day – (or equivalent – see page 82).

## RED MEAT

Maximum of two to three portions per week.

## FISH

Try to eat regularly, especially oily fish.

## FRESH GREEN VEGETABLES

At least once daily, preferably twice.

## SUGAR

Avoid adding sugar to drinks and eating sugary foods.

## EAT SMALL REGULAR SNACKS AND MEALS

See page 37.

## SALT

Avoid adding to food, and try to use a salt substitute in cooking.

## FRESH FRUIT

At least two portions daily.

## WHEAT

Avoid whole wheat products (see details of sensitivities on page 32). It should not be necessary to avoid all grains unless you find that the symptoms mentioned there are persistent.

## WHOLEFOODS

Eat plenty of unprocessed and natural foods.

## EXERCISE

Twenty to thirty minutes per day.

For help with keeping to this regime, see Chapter 10.

# SAMPLE MENUS

Here is a week's worth of sample menus. The starred items will be found in the recipe section. Please use snacks of your choice from p.37.

## DAY 1

Breakfast  2 scrambled eggs on white toast
1 yogurt

Lunch  Smoked mackerel
Minty cabbage salad*
Brown rice

Dinner  Roast chicken
Broccoli
Carrots
Jacket or boiled potatoes

Sweet  Fresh fruit salad*

## DAY 2

Breakfast  Rice Krispies with skimmed milk
Chopped banana and 1 tablespoon linseeds

Lunch       Pizza toast*
            Watercress, fennel and lemon salad*

Dinner      Almond trout*
            Brown rice
            Spinach
            Sweetcorn

Sweet       Apple and tofu cheesecake*


## DAY 3

Breakfast   3 grilled tomatoes on white toast

Lunch       Grilled sardines
            Jacket potato
            Green salad*

Dinner      Gammon steak
            Orange sauce*
            Brown rice
            Carrots
            Broccoli

Sweet       Baked apple*


## DAY 4

Breakfast   Porridge (made with half water and half milk)
            1 chopped banana

Lunch       Nutty sprout stirfry*
            Brown rice

Dinner      Broccoli and sweetcorn plaice*
            Carrots
            Cabbage
            Jacket or boiled potatoes

Sweet       Orange jelly*

## DAY 5

Breakfast    2 slices white toast with sugar-free marmalade

Lunch        Spinach gratin*
             Baked potato

Dinner       Grilled lamb chop
             Gravy
             Courgettes
             Green beans
             Jacket or boiled potatoes

Sweet        Banana and tofu cream*


## DAY 6

Breakfast    Fresh fruit salad*
             1 tablespoon raisins and mixed nuts
             1 yogurt

Lunch        Brown lentil soup*
             2 Ryvitas

Dinner       Halibut fruit*
             Spinach
             Brown rice

Sweet        Slice of pineapple cake*


## DAY 7

Breakfast    2 boiled eggs
             1–2 slices white bread

Lunch        Tuna jacket potato*

Dinner       Grilled lean steak
             Baked nutty onions*
             Broccoli

Grilled tomatoes
Baked or boiled potatoes

Sweet Piece of fresh fruit

# WEEK 2

## DAY 1

Breakfast Yogurt with 1 tablespoon of linseeds
1 chopped banana

Lunch Mushroom with mint soup*
1 slice of white toast

Dinner Chicken with almonds*
Leeks
Broccoli
Brown rice

## DAY 2

Breakfast Cornflakes with skimmed milk
1 chopped apple
1 tablespoon of raisins

Lunch Cooked mussels with lemon juice and black pepper
Brown rice salad*

Dinner Lamb and parsley stew*
Carrots
Spring greens
Mashed potatoes

## DAY 3

Breakfast   1 scrambled egg
1 slice of white toast
2 grilled tomatoes

Lunch   Jacket potato
2 oz grated cheese
Coleslaw salad*

Dinner   Grilled mackerel
Sweetcorn
Broccoli
Sauté potatoes

## DAY 4

Breakfast   Fresh fruit salad*
1 tablespoon linseeds
1 tablespoon mixed nuts

Lunch   Fish soup*
2 rice cakes or 1 slice of white toast

Dinner   Steak and bananas*
Grilled mushrooms
Spinach
Jacket potato

## DAY 5

Breakfast   Rice Krispies with skimmed milk
1 chopped orange

Lunch   Grilled plaice
Tomato sauce*
Spinach salad*

Dinner   Sussex casserole*
Brown rice

## DAY 6

Breakfast  2 boiled eggs
           2 rice cakes with sugar-free jam

Lunch      Cottage cheese
           Beetroot and cabbage salad*
           Potato salad*

Dinner     Prawn provençale*
           Brown rice


## DAY 7

Breakfast  3 grilled tomatoes on white toast
           1 yogurt

Lunch      Jacket potato
           2 grilled sardines
           Bean and sweetcorn salad*

Dinner     Turkey breast with mushroom sauce*
           Spinach
           Leeks
           Sauté potatoes

# 9

# RECOMMENDATIONS AND MENUS FOR SEVERE SUFFERERS

## TEA

Restrict to only one weak cup per day.

## COFFEE

Avoid altogether. Restrict to a maximum of two cups of decaffeinated coffee per day. Preferably substitute altogether (see list and alternative drinks on p. 80).

## COLA-BASED DRINKS

Avoid altogether.

## ALCOHOL

Avoid altogether.

## SMOKING

Try to cut down gradually. It is better to try to reduce your cigarette consumption after your period rather than during your pre-menstrual phase.

## DAIRY

Keep total dairy consumption down to less than half a pint per day (see page 82).

## RED MEAT

Restrict to a maximum of two portions per week, preferably organic or additive-free.

## FISH

Try to eat four to five portions per week, especially oily fish, ie. herring, mackerel, sardines or salmon when in season.

## VEGETABLES AND SALAD GREENS

Eat at least one large serving daily, preferably more, either gently steamed or raw.

## SUGAR

Avoid white or brown sugar and sugary foods.

## SALT

Do not add salt to the cooking or at the table.

## SALTY FOODS

Avoid eating foods with a high salt content.

## FRESH FRUIT

At least two to three portions daily.

## GRAINS

Avoid all wheat, barley, oats, rye and corn (see page 32).

## OILS

Use good-quality polyunsaturated vegetable oils, like sunflower or safflower oils, but try to keep consumption fairly low.

## WHOLEFOODS

Eat plenty of unprocessed and natural foods.

## ADDITIVES

Avoid altogether or greatly restrict listed additives pre-menstrually (see list p.85).

## EXERCISE

Thirty to forty minutes per day.

## OTHER USEFUL ADVICE

1. Eat regular snacks and meals.
2. Plan meals ahead, preferably before you go shopping.

For help with keeping to this regimen, see Chapter 10.


# SAMPLE MENUS

Here are two weeks' worth of sample menus, followed by some vegetarian menus. Please note, white flour can be replaced with rice or potato flour.

# WEEK 1

## DAY 1

Breakfast  Cornflakes
Skimmed milk or apple juice
1 chopped apple
1 tablespoon linseeds

Snack     2–3 oz unsalted nuts or seeds

Lunch     Jacket potato
Sardines
Green salad*

Snack     1 banana

Dinner    Grilled lamb chop with tomato sauce*
Carrots
Fresh greens
Potatoes

Sweet     Orange jelly*

## DAY 2

Breakfast  2–3 rice cakes
Sugar-free jam
Fresh fruit salad*

Snack     1 natural yogurt with 1 tablespoon linseeds

Lunch     Chicken and spinach soup*
French bread

Snack     2–3 oz raw carrot

Dinner    Dutch pork*
Green salad*
Brown rice*

Sweet     Apple custard*

## DAY 3

Breakfast    2 boiled eggs
                    2 rice cakes
                    1 apple

Snack        2–3 oz unsalted mixed nuts

Lunch        Lean ham
                    Jacket potato
                    Coleslaw salad*

Snack        1 banana

Dinner       Haddock Florentine*
                    Brown rice
                    Fresh broccoli
                    Sweetcorn

Sweet        Apple and passion fruit delight*

## DAY 4

Breakfast    Cornflakes
                    Skimmed milk
                    1 banana
                    1 tablespoon linseeds

Snack        1 apple

Lunch        Grilled plaice with mustard sauce*
                    Boiled potatoes
                    Greens
                    Cauliflower

Snack        1 orange

Dinner       Haddock kedgeree*
                    Watercress, fennel and lemon salad*

Sweet        Rhubarb and ginger mousse*

## DAY 5

| | |
|---|---|
| Breakfast | Yogurt with chopped apple<br>1 tablespoon linseeds |
| Snack | 2 rice cakes with sugar-free peanut butter |
| Lunch | Grilled chicken, hot or cold<br>Potato salad*<br>Beetroot cabbage salad* |
| Snack | 2–3 oz unsalted seeds |
| Dinner | Vegetable curry*<br>Brown rice |
| Sweet | Fresh fruit salad* |

## DAY 6

| | |
|---|---|
| Breakfast | Rice Krispies<br>Skimmed milk<br>1 banana<br>1 tablespoon linseeds |
| Snack | 1 apple |
| Lunch | Brown lentil soup*<br>2 rice cakes |
| Snack | 2–3 oz unsalted mixed nuts |
| Dinner | Liver and sweetcorn casserole*<br>Cabbage<br>Grilled mushrooms<br>Baked or boiled potatoes |
| Sweet | Baked apple* |

## DAY 7

Breakfast   Grilled tomatoes
2 egg omelette
Grilled mushrooms
2 rice cakes

Snack   1 banana

Lunch   Sardines
Spinach salad*
Rice salad*

Snack   2 rice cakes with sugar-free jam

Dinner   Hot fruity chicken*
Carrots
Spinach
Jacket potato

Sweet   Fresh mousse*

For the following menus, please add mid-morning, mid-afternoon and mid-evening snacks of your choice from the list on page 37. Fresh fruit or a suitable sweet from the recipe section can be eaten after the main course at dinner.

## WEEK 2

Some white flour has been included in this week for those that find it too difficult to avoid grains altogether.

## DAY 1

Breakfast   Oats, soaked overnight with skimmed milk
Yogurt and chopped banana
1 tablespoon linseeds

Lunch   Pilchards on white toast
Beansprout salad*

Dinner    Roast turkey
          Parsley and lemon stuffing*
          Parsnips
          Cabbage
          Roast potatoes

## DAY 2

Breakfast  1 slice white toast
           Scrambled egg

Lunch     Jacket potato with tuna
          Salad of your choice*

Dinner    Steak and bananas*
          Green beans
          Red cabbage
          Sauté potatoes

## DAY 3

Breakfast  Cornflakes
           Skimmed milk
           Chopped apple
           1 tablespoon linseeds

Lunch     Spinach and avocado salad*
          Brown rice

Dinner    Fish pudding*
          Broccoli
          Grilled tomatoes

## DAY 4

Breakfast  2 Ryvita with sugar-free jam
           1 yogurt with chopped banana
           1 tablespoon linseeds

Lunch        Tomato and black pepper omelette
             Salad of your choice*

Dinner       Red mullet in tomato sauce*
             Green beans
             Sweetcorn
             Boiled potatoes


## DAY 5

Breakfast    Fresh fruit salad*
             1 tablespoon nuts

Lunch        Mushroom and mint soup*
             1 slice white toast

Dinner       Spiced lentil cakes*
             Minty cabbage salad*


## DAY 6

Breakfast    Poached egg on white toast
             Grilled tomatoes

Lunch        Jacket potato
             Baked beans (low salt and sugar)
             2 oz grated cheese

Dinner       Liver kebabs*
             Salad of your choice*
             Brown rice


## DAY 7

Breakfast    Oats soaked overnight with chopped fruit
             Skimmed milk
             1 tablespoon linseeds

Lunch      Bean and carrot soup*
           French bread

Dinner     Pork chops with tomato and mushrooms*
           Spinach
           Carrots
           Boiled potatoes

## SAMPLE DRINKS

Herbal teas                                unlimited

2 cups decaffeinated coffee                maximum

½ glass apple juice/
    orange juice diluted with water   unlimited

Mineral waters                             unlimited

# RECOMMENDATIONS FOR VEGETARIANS AND VEGANS

Vegetarians need to be sure to include a variety of vegetable proteins in their diet as no one vegetable protein contains all the required nutrients. Vegetarian proteins include: nuts, seeds, peas, beans, lentils, whole grain, brown rice, sprouted beans and soya bean products.

Many vegetarians do take good care over their diet but there are some who replace the meat and fish with too much cheese and junk foods. The menus and recipes on page 78 should help you to follow your PMT diet recommendations. They have been designed for vegetarians who are moderate to severe PMT sufferers. If you suffer mild to moderate PMT symptoms, and usually follow a vegetarian diet, you can use the menus as a guideline, and add in wholegrain products, like whole wheat bread, pasta and pastry.

There are also vegans who look after their diets and vegans who do not. It is important to obtain a good specialized vegan recipe book to help you to follow your PMT diet recommendations. You should find that the vegetarian menus will be quite easy to follow with adjustments to meet your vegan regimen.

# SAMPLE VEGETARIAN MENUS

Please add mid-morning, mid-afternoon and mid-evening snacks of your choice from the lists on page 37. For dessert, please have fresh fruit or select a suitable sweet from sweets on page 165.

## DAY 1

Breakfast   Rice Krispies
Apple juice
1 tablespoon linseeds

Lunch   Tofu with minty cabbage salad*
Spicy lentil dressing*

Dinner   Nutty sprout stirfry*
Brown rice

## DAY 2

Breakfast   Live yogurt with chopped banana
1 tablespoon linseeds
2 rice cakes with sugar-free jam

Lunch   Jacket potato with 2 oz cheese
Salad of your choice*

Dinner   Nut and vegetable loaf*
Watercress, fennel and lemon salad*

## DAY 3

Breakfast   2 boiled eggs
1 slice white toast

Lunch   Selection of mixed vegetables and brown rice stir-fried
with 2 tablespoons mixed nuts or beans

Dinner   Spinach gratin*
Jacket potato

## DAY 4

Breakfast    Rice Krispies
             Skimmed milk
             2 rice cakes with sugar-free jam

Lunch        Brown lentil soup*
             French bread

Dinner       Mexican stuffed eggs*
             Salad of your choice*

## DAY 5

Breakfast    Fresh fruit salad*
             Yogurt

Lunch        Chickpea dips*
             1 slice white toast

Dinner       Jacket potato
             Baked nutty onions*
             Spinach

## DAY 6

Breakfast    Cornflakes with chopped apple and orange
             Skimmed milk

Lunch        Jacket potato
             Cottage cheese
             Salad of your choice*

Dinner       Bean and carrot soup*
             Vegetable and dal jackets*

## DAY 7

Breakfast    Grilled tomatoes with white toast

Lunch        Potato and herb omelette*
             Beetroot and cabbage salad*

Dinner       Egg and vegetable bake*
             Brown rice

# 10

# HOW TO FOLLOW
# THE DIET
# RECOMMENDATIONS

This advice, with appropriate adaptations, is also relevant to women who suffer only mild or moderate symptoms.

## TEA

There is one thing to remember when trying herb teas – they will not taste like or replace the need for ordinary tea. Many women find that they are addicted to tea without realizing it until they try to stop. Do bear this in mind when you have your first sip of a herbal or alternative tea and find you do not feel the same satisfaction.

There are many different teas to choose from, which can be bought in one-cup packets to save purchasing a whole box and realizing that, after one cup, it's not the tea for you. Start off making the tea weak and build up the strength as your taste buds adjust. Below are some of the popular ones you might like to try. Experiment with these teas until you find a few that you feel happy to consume on a regular basis.

| Fruity | Herb | Similar to ordinary tea |
|---|---|---|
| Apple and fruit | Fennel | Decaffeinated tea |
| Orange | Camomile | Luakka |
| Orchard Surprise | Nettle | Red bush |
| Kiwi and passion fruit | Matle | |
| Tropical Secret | Peppermint | |
| Sunburst C | | |
| Cranberry Cove | | |
| Rosehip | | |
| Bramble | | |
| Wild forest blackberry | | |
| Raspberry Patch | | |

## COFFEE

The same applies here as with tea – it is very difficult to get the same satisfaction initially. Do try some alternatives such as dandelion coffee (instant, or dandelion root filtered through a coffee machine), chicory or barley cup.

## DECAFFEINATED COFFEE

Caffeine has been well researched and is known to cause symptoms. Although caffeine has been removed from decaffeinated coffee it still contains other chemicals, the effects of which are not fully known. Use the above alternatives for tea or coffee once you have used up your allowance for the day.

## COLA

Cola drinks contain sugar and caffeine. These should be avoided. It is also best to avoid even the diet and low-caffeine alternatives for now also. Try fresh fruit juice with carbonated water or one of the many apple and carbonated water drinks which are available in restaurants and bars.

## ALCOHOL

This is not always very easy to avoid on special occasions or at times of celebration. But nowadays you are no longer considered a party pooper if you do not indulge in an alcoholic beverage – there are now more non-alcoholic or low-alcohol drinks available than ever. More and more people also cater for the drivers and teetottallers in their gatherings. When out, mineral waters such as Perrier and also fruit juice and carbonated water mixes are freely available. The low-alcohol wines and beers should only be drunk once or twice per week.

## SMOKING

We all know that smoking is bad for our health, but it can also worsen some PMT symptoms and reduce certain vitamin levels, particularly vitamin C. This new diet plan should inspire you to cut down drastically and eventually stop. You may need to stabilize your symptoms and adjust to the diet plan before cutting down too drastically.

## DAIRY

Keep your total dairy consumption down to the equivalent of ½ pint of milk per day. This means that you can have 10 fl oz of dairy products per day (2 oz of cheese is equivalent to 4 oz of milk). Dairy products can make PMT symptoms far worse – particularly PMT A symptoms – and can block the uptake of magnesium, which is an important mineral to PMT sufferers. Other calcium-rich foods are almonds, brazil nuts, watercress, figs, broccoli, and parsley.

## MEAT/POULTRY

Keep your red meat consumption down to a maximum of two to three portions per week, and always try to eat lean meats; remove all visible fat before cooking, and remove any skin from poultry. Try to buy additive-free or, better still, organic meat where possible. Pork pies, sausages and mixed meat pies should be avoided for now. Poultry is definitely preferable to too much red meat.

## FISH

Natural fish oils contain important essential fatty acids known as Eicosapentonoic Acid (EPA). Essential fatty acids are important for many body mechanisms, especially in producing hormone-like substances called prostaglandins, which help to balance sex hormones.

It is a myth that fish is fiddly to prepare. A shortage of ideas for making it more exciting seems to be a major reason for women not eating fish more regularly. It can be so quick and easy to prepare – just look at some of the recipes included in that section.


## FRESH GREEN VEGETABLES AND GREENS

Fresh green vegetables supply important nutrients and should be eaten at least once daily, preferably twice. How fresh is fresh? Ideally, you should shop at least twice per week for your vegetables. Keeping them in the fridge will help keep them fresh that bit longer. Try to buy organic vegetables or grow your own in order to lessen your intake of chemicals.

The benefits your body receives from your vegetables depends greatly on how you prepare and cook them. Chopping too small or too finely will allow a greater loss of all the essential vitamins and minerals they contain. Avoid boiling them until soft. Try to change your tastes and those of your family so that you enjoy your vegetables with a little 'bite' or crunch to them. Try using less water, and use a lid on your saucepan; this helps to steam them, which is more economical too. You can also use a metal colander or steamer with a lid, over a saucepan of boiling water. Remember that raw vegetables are very high in nutrients and fibre, so plenty of crunchy salads please.


## SUGAR

Blood sugar levels can be quite a problem for severe sufferers. Avoiding the refined sugars can in fact help your body to correct this problem. You will see from the recipes that sugar is not necessarily needed in 'sweets'. See page 35 for help on sugar craving and a list of alternatives to use.

## REGULAR SNACKS AND MEALS

These help to maintain energy and blood sugar levels, helping to reduce PMT C symptoms, mood swings, irritability and depression. See page 37 for snacks and eating pattern ideas.

## SALT

It can be difficult to stop adding salt when you are cooking for the family. Try to reduce this over a week, and swap to adding a small amount of a salt substitute (avilable from health food shops) instead. It is a good idea not to put the salt pot on the table, so it can not be added to the plate. Using spices, herbs and freshly ground black pepper can reduce the want for the salty taste.

## SALTY FOODS

Pre-packed ham, bacon, processed foods, crisps, salted nuts, tinned fish in brine and so on are all foods that should be kept low but avoided altogether in the two weeks before your period.

## FRESH FRUIT

You should try to eat two or more portions of fruit daily. Always try to keep a fresh supply at home and even at work to use as a snack.

## GRAINS AND WHOLEWHEAT

Avoiding grains and wholewheat can be a difficult task. It is important to ensure that these are substituted in your diet. See page 32 for alternatives and information on how to reintroduce these back into your diet.

## OILS

Always use good-quality vegetable oils for cooking, such as sunflower and safflower seed oils. Cold-pressed oils are also a good source of unsaturated oil for salad dressings.

## WHOLEFOODS

Wholefoods means foods that have not been processed or refined. The term also refers to grains such as whole wheat, barley, oats, millet, rye and oats, which are fine to eat once it is established that there is no sensitivity (see page 31).

## ADDITIVES

Severe PMT sufferers seem to be more sensitive before their period, and therefore more likely to react to certain additives. If you suffer badly it would be best to try and keep the additives below at a very low level in the two weeks before your period.

Azo-dyes E102, E104, E107, E110, E122, E123, E124, E128, E131, E132, E133, E142, E151, E154, E155, E180.
Benzoates E210–E219
Sulphur dioxide and sulphites E220–E227
Nitrites and nitrates E249–E252
Proprionic acid and propionates E280–E283
Anti-oxidants BHA and BHT, E320 and E321
Monosodium glutamate (MSG) and related compounds E621–E623

## PLANNING

When on a restricted diet, planning is all-important. Start not with a negative list of what you cannot have, but with a list of foods that you like that you can have. Try to draw up a rough plan of your meals for the week ahead and for any packed lunches. This will ensure that you have to hand all you need to follow your PMT diet recommendations.

It is usually not possible to cook lunches or follow the sample menus when working full-time, part-time or even just leading a very busy life. This is where planning is very important. If you have access to a work canteen you may be lucky enough to find lunches such as salads, jacket potatoes or chicken and vegetable dishes. Unfortunately this will not always be the case, so home-prepared lunches may be needed at first, especially if following the recommendations for sufferers of severe PMT symptoms.

When preparing your evening meal, give a thought to tomorrow's lunch. You can boil some brown rice and leave it to cool whilst you are cooking. Make an extra portion of salad to be left in the fridge ready to be put into a lunch box in the morning. Here are some suggestions for portable lunches: sardines, tuna, cold chicken, hard-boiled eggs, cold ham, lean beef, prawns, pilchards, tinned salmon, or any cold lean meats can be used with any combination of salads (see page 89).


## EXERCISE

Try twenty to thirty minutes' exercise three times a week, or daily if possible. Any exercise that stimulates the circulation would be great – swimming, squash, cycling, tennis, jogging, aerobics or even a brisk walk.

If you are not used to exercising, start slowly. Join a class or local club – it sometimes helps to make it a social arrangement, so take a friend along. Exercising at home with a tape can be ideal for those with young children, who may like to join in.

Research has shown that regular exercise can be of proven benefit to PMT sufferers. It not only helps to reduce fluid retension but can have a positive effect on endorphin levels. It is difficult to believe that this can help when you are feeling low and exhausted, but exercising regularly can in fact improve fatigue and is a great outlet for irritability and aggressive feelings.

It is now known that exercise will help to keep your bones strong and healthy, which is a sure way to prevent bone thinning and help to reduce the risk of osteoporosis.

# PART III

# THE RECIPES

# 11

# SALADS AND DRESSINGS

Unless organically grown, fruit and vegetables are often sprayed with chemicals. It is, therefore, important that all ingredients are washed well, especially as salads are eaten raw.

## Chicken and Pasta Salad G & W

*Serves 4*

150 g (5 oz) chicken breast fillet
225 g (8 oz) fettucine
2 teaspoons sesame seeds
100 g (4 oz) mange-tout
100 g (4 oz) broccoli cut into florets
1 medium green pepper, cored, seeded and sliced
6 green shallots, chopped

*Dressing*
30 ml (2 tablespoons) lemon juice
15 ml (1 tablespoon) French mustard
1 tablespoon chopped fresh parsley
2 teaspoons grated fresh ginger
30 ml (2 tablespoons) water

1.  Poach, steam or microwave the chicken until tender. Drain, cool and slice finely.

2.  Add the fettucine to a large saucepan of boiling water. Boil rapidly, uncovered, for about 10 minutes or until just tender, and drain. Rinse under cold water and drain again.

3.  Toast the sesame seeds on an oven tray in a moderate oven and leave to cool.

4.  Drop the mange-tout and broccoli into a saucepan of boiling water, return to the boil, drain, place into a bowl of iced water and drain.

5.  To make the dressing, combine all the ingredients in a screw-top jar and shake well.

6.  Place the fettucine on to a serving plate, top with the mange-tout, broccoli, pepper, shallots and chicken, and sprinkle with seasme seeds. Add the dressing just before serving.

# Waldorf Salad G W & Y

*Serves 4*

50 g (2 oz) walnuts
1 head curly endive
2 dessert apples
2 sticks celery
1 tablespoon linseeds

Chop the walnuts, endives, apples and celery, add the linseeds, and mix together.

# Minty Cabbage Salad G W & Y

*Serves 4*

250 g (9 oz) cabbage
1 medium carrot
1 medium green pepper, cored and seeded
1 medium red pepper, cored and seeded

1.  Shred the cabbage, grate the carrot, chop the peppers and mix all the ingredients together.

# Watercress, Fennel and Lemon Salad G W & Y

*Serves 4*

1 large fennel bulb, thinly sliced
1 small bunch watercress, washed and trimmed
1 handful parsley, washed, well dried and finely chopped
freshly ground black pepper
1 tablespoon lemon juice (fresh)
lemon

1. Mix together the fennel, watercress and parsley.

2. Add the black pepper and lemon juice.

3. Thinly slice the lemon, cut each slice into segments and add to the salad.

# Spinach and Avocado Salad G & W

*Serves 4*

40 English spinach leaves
200 g (7 oz) avocado, sliced
12 black olives, stoned and quartered
*Dressing*
10 ml (2 teaspoons) olive oil
15 ml (1 tablespoon) lemon juice (fresh)
1 garlic clove, crushed

1. Remove the thick stalks from the spinach leaves and slice the leaves into bite-size pieces.

2. Combine the spinach, avocado and olives in bowl.

3. Combine the oil, lemon juice and garlic and pour this dressing over the salad.

91

# Beetroot and Cabbage Salad G W & Y

*Serves 4*

175 g (6 oz) firm white cabbage, shredded
175 g (6 oz) red cabbage, grated
175 g (6 oz) carrots, grated
1 small onion, finely chopped
½ red pepper, cored, seeded and chopped
25 g (1 oz) sunflower seeds
175 g (6 oz) raw beetroot, grated

Mix all the ingredients, leaving the beetroot until just before serving.

# Spinach Salad G W & Y

*Serves 4*

100 g (4 oz) courgettes, thinly sliced
75 g (3 oz) carrots, grated
75 g (3 oz) baby turnips, grated
50 g (2 oz) spinach leaves, coarsely chopped
225 g (8 oz) broad beans

Mix all the ingredients together with black pepper and dressing of choice to taste.

# Cole Slaw G & W

*Serves 4*

450 g (1 lb) white cabbage, shredded
100 g (4 oz) carrots grated
1 onion, sliced

2 tablespoons slimmers' mayonnaise *or* dressing *or* slimmers'
   natural yogurt
1 tablespoon finely chopped fresh parsley

Mix all the ingredients together, using the parsley to decorate.

# Beansprout Salad W & Y

*As a side salad serves 4*

175 g (6 oz) beansprouts
100 g (4 oz) red pepper, cored, seeded and sliced
100 g (4 oz) can of sweetcorn, drained
2 dessert apples, grated
4 spring onions, chopped

Mix all the ingredients together with black pepper and dressing to
taste.

# Bean and Sweetcorn Salad W & Y

*As a side salad serves 4*

225 g (8 oz) French beans, cut into 2.5 cm/1 inch lengths
100 g (4 oz) can of sweetcorn, drained
2 small spring onions, sliced
a few sesame seeds

Cook the beans for 5 minutes, drain and cool under cold water.
Drain well, and add the sweetcorn and spring onions with a
sprinkle of sesame seeds.

# Green Salad G W & Y

*Serves 1*

50 g (2 oz) lettuce, chopped
8 slices thinly cut cucumber
½ green pepper, cored, seeded and sliced
50 g (2 oz) watercress

Mix all the ingredients together with black pepper and dressing to taste.

# Brown Rice Salad W & Y

*Serves 2*

100 g (4 oz) cooked brown rice
75 g (3 oz) canned sweetcorn
½ red pepper, cored, seeded and sliced
½ green pepper, cored, seeded and sliced

Mix all the ingredients together with black pepper and dressing to taste.

# Potato Salad G & W

*Serves 2*

225 g (8 oz) boiled potatoes
2 spring onions
2 tablespoons low-calorie dressing
2 teaspoons snipped fresh chives

Chop the potatoes into bite-size pieces. Chop the spring onions. Mix all the ingredients together.

# Bean Salad G W & Y

*As a side salad serves 4*

100 g (4 oz) haricot beans, soaked overnight
100 g (4 oz) chickpeas, soaked overnight
1 bay leaf
2 sprigs of thyme
1 garlic clove, crushed
30 ml (2 tablespoons) cold-pressed olive oil *or* vegetable oil
100 g (4 oz) tined red kidney beans
100 g (4 oz) broad beans
2 tablespoons finely chopped parsley
½ teaspoon cumin seeds, ground
1 medium onion, finely chopped

Drain the haricot beans and chickpeas, and cover with water in a saucepan. Boil for 10 minutes, add the bay leaf and sprigs of thyme, and simmer for 1–1½ hours. Drain and leave to cool. Mix the garlic with the oil and the kidney and broad beans. Pour this over the remaining beans. Add the parsley, cumin seeds and onion.

# Tomato Dressing/Sauce G W & Y

*Serves 4 (2 tablespoons each)*

2 teaspoons olive oil
100 g (4 oz) onion, finely chopped
1 garlic clove, crushed
400 g (14 oz) fresh ripe tomatoes chopped and skin removed,
    *or* 14 oz (400 ml) can plum tomatoes, drained and chopped
½ teaspoon mixed herbs *or* basil
black pepper to taste

Heat the oil, adding the onion and garlic. Cover and cook gently for 5 minutes until the onion is soft. Add the tomatoes and herbs. Cover and cook for 15 minutes. Season with fresh black pepper and cool (if used for salad dressing).

# Spicy Lentil Dressing G W & Y

*Serves 4*

225 g (8 oz) red lentils
600 ml (1 pint) water
2 teaspoons sunflower oil
1 onion, finely chopped
1 garlic clove, crushed
½ teaspoon ginger (ground *or* grated root)
½ teaspoon ground coriander
½ teaspoon ground cumin

1. Place the lentils in a saucepan and cover with the measured water.

2. Bring to the boil and simmer for 20–30 minutes until the water has been absorbed and the lentils are swollen. The lentils should look like a thickish purée.

3. Heat the oil and gently fry the onions, garlic and ginger until lightly brown, for 4–6 minutes.

4. Add the spices and cook further for 1–2 minutes.

5. Add the lentils and cook very gently for 4–5 minutes. Serve hot with rice, or cold with salad.

# Orange and Herb Sauce W

*Serves 4*

2 teaspoons (10 ml) sunflower oil
1 small onion, finely chopped
175 ml (6 fl oz) frozen concentrated orange juice
2 teaspoons chopped tarragon
2 teaspoons chopped parsley
2 teaspoons cornflour
black pepper
1 tablespoon water
1 orange, peeled, segmented, pith removed and chopped

1.  Heat oil and gently fry the onions. Add the orange juice, herbs and black pepper to taste.

2.  Bring to the boil and simmer for 2–3 minutes.

3.  Mix the cornflour with the water and stir into the sauce, bringing slowly to the boil and stirring constantly.

4.  Add the chopped orange segments, heat for 1–2 minutes and serve.

This sauce can be used to complement meat, fish or vegetable dishes, and can be made in larger quantities in advance and frozen.

# 12

# SOUPS

## Mushroom and Mint Soup W

*Serves 4*

4 large potatoes, peeled and coarsely chopped
1 small onion, chopped
900 ml (1½ pints) chicken stock
grated rind *and* juice of 1 lemon
1 tablespoon chopped fresh rosemary
freshly ground black pepper to taste
50 g (2 oz) margarine
225 g (8 oz) mushrooms, sliced
1 tablespoon flour
2 tablespoons finely chopped fresh mint
150 ml (5 fl oz) milk

1. Place the potatoes and onions in a large saucepan and add the stock, lemon rind, juice, rosemary and pepper.

2. Bring the mixture to the boil. Reduce the heat and simmer, stirring occasionally, for 25 minutes or until the vegetables are tender.

3. In a small saucepan, melt the margarine over a low heat. Add the mushrooms and toss them in the margarine until they are thoroughly coated. Cook them slowly, stirring occasionally, for 10 minutes.

4. Sprinkle the flour into the pan and stir it into the mushrooms with a wooden spoon. Set aside for the moment.

5. Remove the potatoes and onion from the stock mixture with a slotted spoon. Purée them in a blender or food processor or push through a sieve with a wooden spoon.

6. Return the purée to the stock mixture. Add the mushrooms.

7. Bring to the boil, stirring constantly. Stir in the mint.

8. Remove from the heat and stir in the milk.

# Brown Lentil Soup G W & Y

*Serves 6–8*

450 g (1 lb) brown lentils
1 litre (1¾ pints) water
2 tablespoons sunflower oil
1 large onion, peeled and finely chopped
2 garlic cloves, crushed
1.4 litres (2½ pints) vegetable stock
1 large carrot, peeled and chopped
2 sticks celery, trimmed and chopped
1 bay leaf
freshly ground black pepper

1. Place the lentils and water in a pan and bring to the boil. Boil for 2 minutes, then remove from the heat and leave to stand for 2 hours, covered. Drain.

2. Heat the oil in a saucepan and lightly brown the onion. Add the garlic and mix well.

3. Stir in the drained lentils, add the stock and bring to the boil.

4. Add the celery, carrots, bay leaf and pepper.

5. Simmer for 45–60 minutes until the lentils are tender, then remove the bay leaf.

6. Half or all the soup can be puréed in a blender or food processor.

# Chilled Tomato Soup G & W

*Serves 4*

450 g (1 lb) tomatoes, skinned, seeded and chopped
100 g (4 oz) cucumber, peeled and chopped
1 clove garlic, crushed
pinch of cayenne
5 ml (1 teaspoon) Worcestershire sauce
1 medium green pepper, cored, seeded and chopped
150 g (5 oz) natural yogurt
chopped fresh parsley to garnish

1. Place the tomatoes, cucumber, garlic, cayenne, Worcestershire sauce, half the green pepper and half the yogurt in a blender or food processor and liquidize until smooth.

2. Chill well.

3. Stir in the remaining green pepper, and the yogurt and sprinkle with parsley before serving.

# Leek and Potato Soup G W & Y

*Serves 4*

1 tablespoon (15 ml) sunflower oil
2 carrots, peeled and sliced
2 leeks, trimmed, washed and sliced
1 large potato, peeled and sliced
freshly ground black pepper
450 ml (¾ pint) vegetable stock
150 ml (¼ pint) skimmed milk
4 small sprigs of watercress to garnish

1. Heat the oil in a saucepan. Add the carrots and leeks, cover and sweat over a low heat for 15 minutes.

2.   Add the potato slices, pepper to taste and 300 ml (½ pint) of the stock. Bring to the boil and simmer until the potatoes are soft.

3.   Liquidize and return to the saucepan, adding the remaining stock and milk. Adjust the seasoning and serve hot or cold with watercress to garnish.

# Bean and Carrot Soup G W & Y

*Serves 4*

15 ml (1 tablespoon) sunflower oil
450 g (1 lb) carrots, peeled and sliced
1 large potato, diced
1 medium onion, chopped
900 ml (1½ pints) water
15 ml (1 tablespoon) tomato puree
good pinch of ground coriander
freshly ground black pepper
425 g (15 oz) can kidney beans, drained
chopped fresh parsley to garnish

1.   Heat the oil in a saucepan, add the vegetables and cook, stirring, for 5 minutes.

2.   Add the water, tomato purée, coriander and pepper to taste and bring to the boil. Lower the heat, cover and simmer for 45 minutes.

3.   Stir in the kidney beans and reheat gently.

4.   Pour into individual soup bowls, garnish with parsley and serve at once.

# Chicken and Spinach Soup G W & Y

*Serves 4*

2 chicken breasts, skinned and each chopped into 8 pieces
600 ml (1 pint) water
2 teaspoons (10 ml) sunflower oil
1 onion, finely chopped
150 g (5 oz) spinach, stalks removed and leaves shredded
600 ml (1 pint) skimmed milk

1. Place the chicken and water in a saucepan, bring to the boil and simmer for 45 minutes.

2. Heat the oil and gently fry the onions for 2 minutes until translucent.

3. Remove the onions with a slotted spoon and add to the chicken and liquid.

4. Add the spinach, season with black pepper to taste, and cook for a further 5 minutes.

5. Add the milk and heat through before serving.

# Fish Soup G & W

*Serves 6*

1.8 litres (3 pints) fish stock
4 medium onions, peeled and finely chopped
freshly ground black pepper to taste
1 tablespoon paprika
900 g (2 lb) filleted white fish cut into 5 cm (2 inch) pieces
1 red chilli chopped finely
1 medium green pepper, seeded and thinly sliced
75 ml (3 fl oz) sour cream

102

1. Bring the fish stock to the boil.

2. Reduce the heat and add the onions, pepper and paprika and stir well.

3. Cover the pan and simmer mixture for 1 hour, or until the onions are soft.

4. Remove the pan from the heat and strain the mixture. Discard any pulp left in the strainer.

5. Add the fish to the strained stock and bring to the boil. Add the chilli, reduce the heat and simmer for 15 to 20 minutes or until the fish flakes easily when tested with a fork.

6. Transfer the soup to a warmed tureen. Stir in the sour cream and serve immediately.

# 13

# FISH

## Tuna Jackets w

*Serves 4*

15 ml (1 tablespoon) sunflower oil
1 red *and* 1 yellow *and* 1 green pepper, cored, seeded and diced
4 tablespoons (60 ml) white wine vinegar
30 ml (2 tablespoons) wholegrain mustard
200 g (7 oz) can tuna in oil, drained and flaked
100 g (4 oz) can sweetcorn, drained
4 hot baked potatoes
fresh black pepper

1.  Heat the oil, add the diced peppers and sauté for 5 minutes. Add the vinegar and mustard and cook for 5 minutes, stirring.

2.  Stir in the flaked tuna and sweetcorn.

3.  Cut the tops off the potatoes and scoop out the centres. Chop the potato and stir it into half the pepper relish mixture. Season with black pepper to taste.

4.  Spoon the potato mixture back into the potato jackets. Serve the remaining relish separately.

# Prawn Provençale G W & Y

## Serves 4

50 g (2 oz) margarine
30 ml (2 tablespoons) olive oil
4 shallots, finely chopped
1 garlic clove, crushed (optional)
6 tomatoes, blanched, peeled and chopped
50 g (2 oz) tomato purée
1 teaspoon dried thyme
1 pinch dried basil
black pepper to taste
675 g (1½ lbs) cooked peeled prawns

1.  In a large frying-pan, heat the margarine with the oil. Add the shallots and garlic and fry them for 4 minutes.

2.  Add the tomatoes, tomato purée, thyme, basil and pepper to taste. Cover the pan, reduce the heat to low and simmer for 20 minutes. Stir in the prawns and cook uncovered for a further 4 minutes.

3.  Remove from heat and serve at once.

# Tuna Surprise G & W

## Serves 2–3

15 ml (1 tablespoon) sunflower oil
1 large onion, chopped
1 garlic clove, chopped
½ teaspoon curry powder
225 g (8 oz) can tomatoes
225 g (8 oz) can tuna fish in oil, drained well
1 teaspoon dried basil
2 tablespoons sultanas or seedless raisins
freshly ground black pepper

1. In a medium saucepan, heat the oil, add the onion and garlic and fry for 5 minutes or until the onion is soft and translucent.

2. Stir in the curry powder and add the tomatoes with their juice, tuna, basil, sultanas and pepper to taste.

3. Bring to the boil, reduce the heat to low and simmer gently for 10 minutes.

4. Serve with rice, paste or potatoes, and vegetables.

# Japanese Sardines G & W

*Serves 4*

100 ml (4 fl oz) soy sauce
50 ml (2 fl oz) vinegar
30 ml (2 tablespoons) lemon juice
25 g (1 oz) fresh root ginger, peeled and chopped
2 garlic cloves, crushed
450 g (1 lb) fresh sardines, washed thoroughly in cold water and dried

1. In a small mixing bowl, combine the soy sauce, vinegar, lemon juice, ginger and garlic.

2. Arrange the sardines in a shallow baking dish and pour the soy sauce mixture over them. Leave in a cool place to marinate for 1½–2 hours.

3. Remove the sardines from the marinade and discard the marinade.

4. Grill for 3–5 minutes or longer, depending on the size, and turning once. Serve immediately.

# Halibut Fruit G W & Y

*Serves 2*

grated rind and juice of 2 oranges *and* 1 lemon, *plus* 1 orange,
    peeled, segmented and skinned, *plus* extra slices for garnish
2 halibut steaks, cut in half

1.  Place the grated rinds into an ovenproof dish with the juices.
    Add the fish and baste well. This can be left to marinade for
    1–6 hours, turning occasionally.

2.  Cover the dish with foil and cook in a pre-heated oven at
    180°C (350°F) gas mark 4 for 10 minutes.

3.  Add the orange segments and cook for a further 10 minutes.

4.  Garnish with a slice of lemon and orange.

# Almond Trout G W & Y

*Serves 4*

4 trout, cleaned, with heads and tails intact
freshly ground black pepper
juice of 1 lemon
25 g (1 oz) margarine
50 g (2 oz) flaked almonds
4 sprigs parsley to garnish

1.  Season the fish with pepper and lemon juice.

2.  Melt the margarine and lightly brush the fish.

3.  Place the fish under a hot grill and cook for 6 minutes each
    side.

4.  Brush one side again lightly with melted margarine and ar-
    range almonds over the fish. Grill again for 1 minute or until
    the almonds start to brown.

5.  Garnish with parsley and serve.

# Plaice with Yogurt and Nuts W & Y

## Serves 4

675 g (1½ lb) plaice fillets
2 bananas, sliced
75 g (3 oz) unsalted peanuts *plus* 25 g (1 oz) peanuts, crushed,
  for garnish
*Sauce*
50 g (2 oz) margarine
50 g (2 oz) plain flour
300 ml (½ pint) milk
45 ml (3 tablespoons) natural yogurt
freshly ground black pepper

1.  Place the fish in a greased, shallow ovenproof dish, cover and cook in a pre-heated oven at 180°C (350°F) gas mark 4 for 10 minutes.

2.  Remove the fish from the oven and arrange the banana and nuts over the fish.

3.  Melt the margarine in a pan and stir in the flour. Cook for 1 minute and gradually add the milk until the sauce thickens. Remove from the heat and add the yogurt.

4.  Season the fish with pepper to taste.

5.  Pour the sauce over the fish and return to the oven for 15 minutes.

6.  Garnish with the finely chopped nuts.

# Broccoli and Sweetcorn Stuffed Plaice W & Y

*Serves 4*

4 plaice fillets
freshly ground black pepper
*Stuffing*
50 g (2 oz) broccoli tops
50 g (2 oz) cooked brown rice
25 g (1 oz) canned sweetcorn
15 ml (1 tablespoon) lemon juice (fresh)
4 slices lemon to garnish

1. Pre-heat the oven to 180°C (350°F) gas mark 4.

2. Skin the plaice fillets and sprinkle them with black pepper to taste.

3. Cook the broccoli tops, drain well and chop.

4. Place the broccoli, rice and sweetcorn into a bowl and mix well with a little lemon juice.

5. Divide the mixture between the 4 plaice fillets, roll up and secure with a cocktail stick.

6. Place in an ovenproof dish, cover and bake for 25–30 minutes, until the fish is tender.

7. Place on a warm plate, remove the cocktail sticks, and garnish with a slice of lemon to serve.

# Mackerel with Lemon Stuffing G W & Y

*Serves 4*

Four 175 g (6 oz) mackerel, split and boned
juice of half a lemon
freshly ground black pepper
3 tablespoons water
4 slices lemon to garnish

*Stuffing*
10 ml (2 teaspoons) sunflower oil
1 small onion, finely chopped
125 g (4 oz) cooked brown rice
finely grated rind *and* juice of a lemon
1 tablespoon freshly chopped parsley
1 small egg (size 4), beaten

1.  Pre-heat the oven to 160°C (325°F) gas mark 3.

2.  First prepare the stuffing. Heat the oil in a pan, add the onions and cook for 5 minutes or until golden.

3.  Transfer to a mixing bowl and combine with the remaining stuffing ingredients.

4.  Place the mackerel on a flat surface and sprinkle the flesh with lemon juice and black pepper.

5.  Spoon the stuffing into the fish and reshape.

6.  Place in an ovenproof dish and add the 3 tablespoons of water.

7.  Cover and poach for 15–20 minutes.

8.  Garnish with the lemon slices.

# Haddock Florentine G W & Y

*Serves 2*

2 × 150 g (5 oz) haddock portions
225 g (8 oz) fresh or frozen spinach, defrosted and drained
30 ml (2 tablespoons) lemon juice (fresh)
2 slices lemon

1. Pre-heat the oven to 220°C (420°F) gas mark 5.

2. Place each haddock portion on to a piece of aluminium foil.

3. Cover each portion with half the spinach and 1 tablespoon of lemon juice and wrap in the foil.

4. Bake for 20–30 minutes.

5. Remove the foil and serve with a slice of lemon to garnish.

# Haddock Kedgeree G W & Y

*Serves 2*

175 g (6 oz) unsmoked haddock, filleted and skinned
75 g (3 oz) brown rice
1 hard-boiled egg, chopped
½ green pepper, cored, seeded and chopped
2 tablespoons low-fat natural yogurt
1 small onion, finely chopped
1 sprig parsley, chopped
freshly ground black pepper to taste
2 slices lemon

1. Cover the fish with water in a shallow pan. Heat gently and poach for about 8–10 minutes.

2. Remove the fish and flake.

3. Boil the rice in the poaching water left in the pan for about 10 minutes. See cooking instructions on the rice packet. You may need to add extra water.

4.  Drain the rice, stir in the fish, egg, green pepper, yogurt, onion, and parsley and mix well. Heat gently, stirring all the time.

5.  Season with pepper and serve garnished with lemon.

# Red Mullet in Tomato Sauce G W & Y

*Serves 6*

60 ml (4 tablespoons) sunflower oil
1.1 kg (2½ lb) tomatoes, blanched, peeled, seeded and
    coarsely chopped
1 teaspoon dried thyme
1 bay leaf
1 teaspoon freshly ground black pepper
225 g (8 oz) black olives, stoned
2 lemons, cut into 12 slices
6 medium red mullet, cleaned and scaled but with heads and
    tails left on

1.  In a large frying pan heat the oil. Add the tomatoes, thyme, bay leaf and pepper. Reduce the heat to low and cook, stirring occasionally, for 15–20 minutes or until the sauce is very thick.

2.  Add the olives and lemon slices and stir well. Transfer half the mixture to another frying pan.

3.  Place 3 fish in each pan and turn them over in the sauce until they are well coated.

4.  Cover the pans and cook, turning the fish occasionally, for 15–20 minutes or until the flesh flakes easily when it is tested with a fork.

5.  Discard the bay leaf and serve.

# Fish Stew with Peppers G W & Y

## Serves 4

30 ml (2 tablespoons) sunflower oil
450 g (1 lb) canned peeled tomatoes
1 red chilli, seeded and finely chopped
2 green peppers, cored, seeded and sliced
2 medium onions, finely chopped
3 garlic cloves, crushed
50 ml (2 fl oz) dry white wine (avoid on a yeast-free diet)
1 teaspoon dried thyme
1 bay leaf
900 g (2 lb) sole fillets, cut into 2.5 cm (1 inch) cubes
450 g (1 lb) small new potatoes, scrubbed, cooked until just
tender and kept warm

1. In an ovenproof dish heat the oil and add the tomatoes, including the juice, and the chilli. Stirring occasionally, cook for 15 minutes or until the mixture is thick.

2. Stir in the green peppers, onions, garlic, wine, thyme, bay leaf and fish cubes. Cover the dish, reduce the heat to low, and cook for 10 minutes, stirring occasionally.

3. Add the potatoes and turn them over in the fish mixture. Cover again and cook for a further 5 minutes, until the fish flakes easily when tested with a fork.

4. Discard the bay leaf and serve at once.

# Fish Pudding W & Y

*Serves 4*

100 g (4 oz) margarine
25 g (1 oz) fine dry white breadcrumbs
2 tablespoons flour
1 teaspoon cornflour
300 ml (10 fl oz) milk
450 g (1 lb) halibut steaks, poached, skinned, boned and
  flaked
225 g (8 oz) cod fillets, poached, skinned, boned and flaked
1 teaspoon freshly ground black pepper
pinch cayenne
pinch dried dill
finely grated rind of 1 lemon
4 eggs, separated

1. Pre-heat the oven to 180°C (350°F) gas mark 4.

2. Grease a 1.7 litre (3 pint) soufflé or baking dish with some of
   the margarine. Sprinkle in the breadcrumbs. Press them lightly
   on the bottom and sides of the dish.

3. In a pan melt half the remaining margarine. Stir in the flour
   and cornflour with a wooden spoon to make a smooth paste.
   Gradually stir in the milk, avoiding the sauce turning lumpy.

4. Cook the sauce for 2–3 minutes, stirring constantly, until it
   thickens. Do not allow the sauce to boil.

5. Remove the pan from the heat and set aside. Beat the fish and
   the remaining margarine in a large mixing bowl until the
   mixture is well combined. Stir in the sauce. Beat in the black
   pepper, cayenne, dill, lemon rind and egg yolks.

6. In a separate bowl, beat the egg whites with a rotary whisk
   until they form stiff peaks. Carefully fold the egg whites into
   the fish mixture. Spoon the mixture into the prepared dish and
   place in a roasting tin half filled with hot water.

7. Place the tin in the centre of the oven and bake the pudding
   for 45–50 minutes or until it is golden brown on top.

8.   Remove the tin from the oven and lift out the dish. Serve the pudding immediately.

# Salmon Potato Cakes G W & Y

*Serves 4*

450 g (1 lb) can salmon
200 g (7 oz) potatoes, coarsely grated
1 egg, lightly beaten
3 green shallots, sliced
10 ml (2 teaspoons) vegetable oil
*Sauce*
1 teaspoon lemon juice (fresh)
13 g (½ oz) sachet vegetable soup mix

1.   Drain the salmon and reserve the liquid. Remove bones and skin from salmon.

2.   Place the salmon in a bowl and mix in the potatoes, egg and shallots. Divide the mixture into 8 portions and pat into the desired shape.

3.   For the sauce, combine the reserved salmon liquid and enough water to measure 100 ml (4 fl oz). Place in a small saucepan with the lemon juice and bring to the boil. Then stir in the soup mix.

4.   Heat the oil in a frying pan, add the cakes and fry on each side until golden brown and firm. Serve with the sauce.

# Fish Moussaka W & Y

## Serves 4

2 large aubergines
175 ml (6 fl oz) vegetable oil
30 ml (2 tablespoons) sunflower oil
2 small onions, finely chopped
225 g (8 oz) cod fillets, cooked, skinned and flaked
450 g (1 lb) halibut steaks, cooked, skinned and flaked
400 g (14 oz) canned tomatoes, chopped
pinch of cayenne
pinch of dried thyme
1 teaspoon dried dill
freshly ground black pepper to taste
1 tablespoon paprika
100 g (4 oz) Cheddar cheese, grated.

*Sauce*
25 g (1 oz) margarine
2 tablespoons flour
350 ml (12 fl oz) milk
4 egg yolks
15 ml (1 tablespoon) lemon juice

1. Pre-heat the oven to 190°C (375°F) gas mark 5.

2. Cut the aubergines into slices.

3. In a large frying pan heat 50 ml (2 fl oz) of the vegetable oil, over a moderate heat. Add about one-third of the aubergine slices and fry for 3–4 minutes on each side or until they are golden brown.

4. Remove with a spatula and allow to drain on kitchen paper. Fry the remaining slices in the same way, adding more oil as necessary. Set aside.

5. Heat the sunflower oil over a moderate heat. Add the onions and cook, stirring occasionally, for 5–7 minutes.

6.  Stir in the fish, tomatoes and their juice, cayenne, thyme, dill, pepper and paprika. Cook, stirring frequently, for 3 minutes. Remove the pan from the heat and set aside.

7.  Arrange one-third of the aubergine on the bottom of an ovenproof dish. Spoon over them half the fish and tomato mixture. Sprinkle half the cheese over the top.

8.  Cover with another third of the aubergine slices and cover that with the remaining fish and tomato mixture. Sprinkle remaining cheese over the top.

9.  Cover with the remaining aubergine slices. Set aside.

10. To make the sauce, melt the margarine in a medium saucepan over a moderate heat.

11. Remove the pan from the heat and, with a wooden spoon, stir in the flour to make a smooth paste.

12. Gradually stir in the milk, being careful to avoid lumps.

13. Return the pan to the heat and cook, stirring constantly, for 2–3 minutes until it is very thick and smooth.

14. Cool the sauce. When cooled, beat in the egg yolks. Stir in the lemon juice.

15. Pour the sauce over the aubergine slices to cover them completely.

16. Place the dish in the centre of the oven and bake for 35–40 minutes or until the top is golden brown. Serve immediately.

# Fisherman's Pie W

## Serves 4

450 g (1 lb) potatoes
350 g (12 oz) haddock *or* cod fillet
100 g (4 oz) mushrooms
227 g (8 oz) can tinned tomatoes
freshly ground black pepper
10 ml (2 teaspoons) oil
1 medium onion, chopped
50 g (2 oz) margarine
50 g (2 oz) plain flour
200 ml (⅓ pint) skimmed milk
100 g (4 oz) peeled prawns (optional)
1 medium tomato, thinly sliced

1.  Pre-heat the oven to 180°C (350°F) gas mark 4.

2.  Boil and mash the potatoes.

3.  Cut the fish into large pieces and place them in a casserole dish. Cover with the mushrooms, tomatoes and a little of the tomato juice from the can, and season with pepper to taste.

4.  Heat the oil and gently fry the onions.

5.  Melt the margarine in a saucepan, add the flour and stir for 1 minute. Gradually add the milk and stir until the sauce thickens. Stir in the cooked onions.

6.  Add the prawns to the saucepan and pour the sauce over the fish.

7.  Cover with the mashed potato and arrange the sliced tomato over the top.

8.  Cook for 30 minutes until golden.

# 14

# MEAT

## Steaks with Mixed Herbs G & W

*Serves 4*

4 rump steaks about 2 cm (¾ inch) thick
freshly ground black pepper to taste
50 g (2 oz) margarine
2 tablespoons freshly chopped parsley
1 tablespoon freshly chopped tarragon
1 tablespoon freshly chopped chives
50 g (2 oz) finely chopped mushrooms
50 ml (2 fl oz) milk

1.  Place the steaks on a board and sprinkle with pepper. Set aside.

2.  Melt the margarine in a large frying pan over a moderate heat. Add the steaks, parsley, tarragon, chives and mushrooms and fry for 2 minutes on each side, stirring constantly.

3.  Reduce the heat and cook for a further 2 minutes on each side. Double the time for well-done steaks.

4.  Remove the steaks from the pan and transfer to a warmed serving dish. Keep them hot while you make the sauce.

5.  Pour the milk into the pan and cook for 2 minutes, stirring constantly until the mixture is hot but not boiling.

6.  Remove the pan from the heat, pour the sauce over the steaks and serve immediately.

# Steak and Bananas W & Y

*Serves 6*

1 egg, well beaten
75 g (3 oz) fresh white breadcrumbs
6 firm bananas, peeled and cut into 1.5 cm (½ inch) slices
50 g (2 oz) margarine
6 fillet steaks
15 ml (1 tablespoon) vegetable oil
freshly ground black pepper to taste
225 ml (8 fl oz) horseradish sauce (if not on low-yeast diet)

1. Pre-heat the grill on high.

2. Pour the egg into a shallow dish and place the breadcrumbs on a plate.

3. Dip the banana slices in the egg and then coat them with the breadcrumbs. Set aside.

4. In a large frying pan melt the margarine over a moderate heat and fry the banana slices for 3 minutes, turning once.

5. Remove from the pan with a slotted spoon and drain excess fat on kitchen paper. Keep the bananas hot while you cook the steaks.

6. Brush the steaks with the oil and sprinkle with pepper. Place the steaks on a rack under the grill and grill for 2 minutes each side. Reduce the heat and cook for a further 2 minutes each side. Double the cooking time for well-done steaks.

7. Transfer the steaks to a warmed serving dish, arrange the bananas around them and serve immediately with the horseradish sauce.

# Sussex Casserole W & Y

*Serves 4–5*

900 g (2 lb) potatoes, peeled and thickly sliced
900 g (2 lb) lean braising steak, cut into 2.5 cm (1 inch) cubes
2 medium size onions, peeled and finely chopped
6 sticks celery, trimmed and chopped
450 g (1 lb) pickling onions
8 green olives, stoned
freshly ground black pepper to taste
5 ml (1 teaspoon) grated nutmeg
4 whole cloves (optional)
1 tablespoon apple juice
450 ml (1 pint) vegetable stock
1 tablespoon cornflour dissolved in water

1.  Pre-heat the oven to 180°C (350°F) gas mark 4.

2.  Cover the bottom of an ovenproof casserole with half of the potato slices.

3.  Arrange half the steak cubes on top and cover with the onions, celery, pickling onions and olives. Sprinkle with black pepper and nutmeg.

4.  Add the cloves (optional).

5.  Cover with remaining steak and potatoes.

6.  Mix the apple juice, stock and cornflour mixture.

7.  Pour over the meat, vegetables and potato. Cover and cook for 2½ hours. Remove the lid and increase the heat to 200°C (400°F) gas mark 6 for a further 30 minutes, or until the potatoes are tender and golden brown. Remove from the oven and serve at once. Remove cloves.

# Beef and Bean Casserole G W & Y

## Serves 4

450 g (1 lb) black-eyed beans, soaked for 12 hours
1.4 litres (2½ pints) cold water
15 ml (1 tablespoon) sunflower oil
2 large onions, finely chopped
2 garlic cloves, crushed
900 g (2 lb) stewing beef, cut into 2.5 cm (1 inch) cubes
1 bay leaf
½ teaspoon dried marjoram
4 large tomatoes, blanched, peeled and sliced
175 ml (6 fl oz) vegetable stock
freshly ground black pepper
1 green pepper, cored, seeded and chopped

1. Pre-heat the oven to 180°C (350°F) gas mark 4.

2. Drain the beans, add fresh water and bring to the boil. Reduce the heat and simmer for 1½ hours, or until the beans are tender.

3. Drain the beans, reserving all the liquid.

4. Heat the oil and gently fry the onions and garlic for 5 minutes, stirring occasionally. Remove from the pan with a slotted spoon and place to one side.

5. Raise the heat, add the cubes of beef and cook until browned all over. Remove from the pan and place in an ovenproof dish.

6. Add to the beef the onions, garlic, bay leaf, marjoram, tomatoes and beef stock, and season with fresh black pepper to taste.

7. Cover and cook for 2 hours.

8. Remove the casserole from the oven and add the beans, chopped pepper and reserved liquid.

9. Return to the oven and cook for a further hour, stirring occasionally.

# Pork Chops with Tomatoes and Mushrooms G & W

*Serves 4*

4 boned loin pork chops
30 ml (2 tablespoons) vegetable oil
1 teaspoon dried thyme
1 tablespoon margarine
100 g (4 oz) mushrooms, sliced
400 g (14 oz) canned tomatoes, chopped
1 teaspoon dried sage
1 tablespoon chopped fresh parsley
freshly ground black pepper to taste

1. Pre-heat the grill on a high heat.

2. Brush the chops with the oil. Sprinkle the thyme and pepper over them. Lay the chops on the rack in the grill pan.

3. Grill the chops for 5 minutes each side. Reduce the heat and cook for 15–20 minutes on each side, depending on the thickness of the chops, or until they are thoroughly cooked.

4. Meanwhile make the sauce. In a large frying pan, melt the margarine over a moderate heat. Add the mushrooms and fry for 3 minutes, stirring occasionally.

5. Add the tomatoes with their juice, the sage, parsley and pepper to taste.

6. Cover the pan and cook on a low heat for 15 minutes.

7. Remove the chops from the grill and arrange in a warmed serving dish. Spoon the sauce over the meat and serve immediately.

# Pork with Cranberry Sauce w

## Serves 4

4 large boned pork chops, trimmed of excess fat
25 g (1 oz) seasoned flour made with 25 g (1 oz) white flour,
    pinch of cayenne and ½ teaspoon dried rosemary
1 tablespoon margarine
15 ml (1 tablespoon) vegetable oil
60 ml (4 tablespoons) canned cranberries
150 ml (5 fl oz) dry white wine
freshly ground black pepper to taste
30 ml (2 tablespoons) milk

1.  Dip the chops in the seasoned flour and coat thoroughly on all sides. Shake off any excess flour.

2.  Melt the margarine with the oil in a large frying pan. Add the pork chops and fry for 5 minutes each side, or until they are well browned.

3.  Reduce the heat and continue cooking the chops for 20–30 minutes or until they are thoroughly cooked and tender.

4.  Transfer the chops to a warmed serving dish and keep the chops hot whilst you make the sauce.

5.  Remove the frying pan from the heat and pour off all the fat except 1 tablespoon.

6.  Return the pan to the heat and stir in the cranberries, wine and pepper. Bring to the boil. Cook the sauce for 5 minutes, stirring constantly.

7.  Stir in the milk and pour the sauce over the chops. Serve immediately.

# Dutch Pork w

## Serves 6–8

450 g (1 lb) loin pork, boned and trimmed of excess fat
1 teaspoon black pepper
½ teaspoon mustard
2 teaspoons dried sage
2 tablespoons raisins
1 large cooking apple, peeled, cored and thinly sliced
15 ml (1 tablespoon) apple juice
50 g (2 oz) margarine
700 g (25 oz) canned apricots in fruit juice, drained and juice
   reserved
1½ teaspoons cornflour, dissolved in water

1.  Pre-heat the oven to 180°C (350°F) gas mark 4.

2.  Place the loin of pork on a work surface and rub with the pepper, mustard and sage.

3.  Lay the meat fat side down and sprinkle with half the raisins. Cover the raisins with apple slices and sprinkle with the remaining raisins.

4.  Roll the meat and tie with string at 2.5 cm (1 inch) intervals.

5.  In a large roasting tin, melt the margarine over a moderate heat. Place the pork in the tin and fry, turning the meat from time to time for 8 minutes or until it is browned all over.

6.  Remove the roasting tin from the heat and place in the centre of the oven. Roast the meat, basting occasionally, for 2½ hours or until it is tender and the juices run clear when the meat is pierced with a sharp knife.

7.  Fifteen minutes before the meat is cooked, pre-heat the grill on a high heat. Arrange the apricots in a heatproof dish, sprinkle with the apple juice and place under the grill for 5–6 minutes until the tops of the apricots are pale brown. Remove the dish and keep warm.

8. Remove the roasting tin from the oven and transfer the pork to a carving dish. Remove the string from the meat and arrange the apricots around the pork. Keep warm while you prepare the sauce.

9. Pour off most of the pork fat from the tin, leaving about 3 tablespoons. Place the tin over a moderate heat and pour in the reserved apricot juice. Stir in the cornflour mixture and bring the sauce to the boil, stirring constantly.

10. Remove the sauce from the heat and strain the sauce into a warmed sauce boat. Serve immediately with the meat.

# Piquant Pork Chops w

*Serves 4*

4 pork chops, trimmed of excess fat
2 garlic cloves, crushed
½ teaspoon dried basil
50 ml (2 fl oz) sunflower oil
100 ml (4 fl oz) dry cider
30 ml (2 tablespoons) wine vinegar
15 ml (1 tablespoon) apple juice
½ teaspoon freshly ground black pepper
½ teaspoon cayenne
3 large carrots, peeled and sliced on the diagonal
½ cucumber, sliced on the diagonal
1 green pepper, cored, seeded and cut into strips
1 tablespoon cornflour, dissolved in 4 tablespoons of water

1. Rub the pork chops all over with the garlic and basil. Set aside.

2. In a large frying pan heat the oil and fry the chops for 5 minutes on each side. Cover the pan, reduce the heat to low and cook the chops for 30 minutes.

3. Transfer the chops to a plate and set aside. Pour off all but 2 tablespoons of the juice and return to a moderate heat.

4. Stir in the cider, vinegar, apple juice, pepper and cayenne and bring the sauce to the boil, stirring constantly.

5. Mix in the vegetables, cover the pan and cook for 2 minutes.

6. Remove the pan from the heat and stir in the cornflour mixture. Return to the heat and, stirring constantly, cook for 1 minute until the sauce is thick and translucent.

7. Return the chops to the pan and baste well with the sauce. Cover the pan and simmer for 5 minutes.

8. Transfer the chops to a warm serving dish and pour the sauce and vegetables over them.

# Herb-Baked Gammon W & Y

*Serves 4*

1.4 kg (3 lb) middle leg of gammon, washed, soaked in cold
   water overnight and drained
2 tablespoons chopped fresh parsley
1 teaspoon dried basil
1 tablespoon chopped mint
1 teaspoon dried thyme
1 tablespoon chopped fresh chives
1 tablespoon grated lemon rind
1 teaspoon grated orange rind
freshly ground black pepper to taste
50 g (2 oz) fresh white breadcrumbs
1 egg, lightly beaten

1. Pre-heat the oven to 170°C (325°F) gas mark 3.

2. Cover the gammon in foil, twisting the edges, and place on a rack in a roasting tin half filled with water.

3. Bake for 2½ hours, turning the gammon over halfway through.

4. Remove the gammon and allow to rest in foil for 30 minutes. (Keep the oven on.)

5. In a bowl, mix together the remaining ingredients and put to one side.

6. Using a sharp knife, remove most of the rind and fat from the gammon joint.

7. Press the herb mixture firmly into the joint with your fingertips.

8. Bake for a further 10–15 minutes. Serve either immediately, or cold with salad.

# Lamb and Parsley Stew W & Y

*Serves 4*

30 ml (2 tablespoons) vegetable oil
1 garlic clove crushed (optional)
1 large onion, sliced
450 g (3 lb) boned shoulder of lamb, trimmed of excess fat and cubed
600 ml (1 pint) of vegetable stock
4 tablespoons of finely chopped freshly parsley
1 bay leaf
6 large tomatoes, blanched, peeled and chopped
4 tablespoons of tomato purée
2 carrots scraped and sliced
1 x 225 g (8 oz) can of red kidney beans, drained
1 tablespoon cornflour dissolved in 2 tablespoons of water

1. Heat the oil in a medium-sized flameproof casserole and then add the garlic, onions and lamb cubes. Fry for 7 to 8 minutes, stirring constantly until the meat is brown on all sides.

2. Stir in the stock, parsley, bay leaf, tomatoes, tomato purée, carrots and bring to the boil. Cover and simmer for 1 hour.

3. Add the kidney beans and cornflour mixture to the stew and stir well. Simmer for 15 minutes, or until the lamb is tender and the sauce is thick. Remove the bay leaf and serve immediately.

# Lamb and Apricot Pilaff G & W

## Serves 4

30 ml (2 tablespoons) sunflower oil
1 medium onion, thinly sliced
700 g (1½ lb) boned leg of lamb, cut into 2.5 cm (1 inch)
  cubes
75 g (3 oz) dried apricots, soaked overnight, drained and
  halved
3 tablespoons raisins
½ teaspoon ground cinnamon
freshly ground black pepper
900 ml (1½ pints) water
225 g (8 oz) long-grain rice, washed, soaked in cold water for
  30 minutes and drained

1.  Heat the oil in a frying pan, add the onion and cook for about
    5 minutes, until translucent but not brown.

2.  Add the lamb and cook, stirring and turning occasionally, for
    5–8 minutes, or until it is lightly browned all over. Stir in the
    apricots, raisins, cinnamon and pepper.

3.  Pour in 450 ml (6 fl oz) of the water and bring to the boil,
    stirring occasionally. Reduce the heat to low, cover the pan
    and simmer the meat for 1–1¼ hours, or until the meat is
    tender when pierced with the point of a sharp knife.

4.  Cook the rice in the usual way, using the remaining water.

5.  Pre-heat the oven to 180°C (350°F) gas mark 4.

6.  Place one-third of the rice in a medium ovenproof casserole.
    Cover with a layer of one-third of the meat mixture, then top
    with another one-third of the rice. Continue to make layers in
    this manner until all the ingredients have been used up,
    finishing with a layer of rice. Cover the casserole and bake for
    50 minutes. Serve immediately.

# Lamb in a Spicy Yogurt Sauce G W & Y

*Serves 4*

225 ml (8 fl oz) water
15 ml (1 tablespoon) olive oil
3 onions, sliced
900 g (2 lb) leg of lamb, boned and cut into 1.8 cm (¾ inch) cubes
freshly ground black pepper
2 garlic cloves, crushed
1 teaspoon chopped fresh parsley
600 ml (1 pint) yogurt
1 tablespoon cornflour mixed to a paste with 2 teaspoons water
1 teaspoon grated lemon rind
1 tablespoon chopped fresh coriander leaves (dried can be used)

1. In a large saucepan, bring the water and oil to the boil over moderate heat.

2. Add the onions, lamb, pepper, garlic and parsley. Cover the pan tightly, reduce the heat to low and simmer for 1¼ hours or until the lamb is very tender and the liquid has reduced by about two-thirds of its original quantity.

3. In a medium saucepan, heat the yogurt and cornflour mixture over a moderate heat, stirring constantly. Reduce the heat to very low and cook for 8 minutes or until it has reduced by half its original quantity.

4. Add the yogurt mixture and the lemon rind to the lamb mixture, stir well and simmer, uncovered, for 15 minutes.

5. Add the coriander and serve with a crisp salad and boiled rice.

# Lamb Chops with Rosemary G W & Y

*Serves 4*

45 ml (3 tablespoons) olive oil
30 ml (2 tablespoons) lemon juice (fresh)
freshly ground black pepper
2 teaspoons dried rosemary
1 garlic clove, crushed
4 thick lamb chops

1.  In a medium-sized shallow mixing bowl combine the oil, lemon juice, pepper to taste, rosemary and garlic.

2.  Place the lamb chops in the marinade and baste them well. Set aside in a cool place and marinate for 1–2 hours, basting frequently.

3.  Pre-heat the grill to high. Place the lamb chops on the grill rack. Reserve the marinade. Grill the chops for 2 minutes on each side, basting them frequently with the marinade, or until they are tender when pierced with the point of a sharp knife.

4.  Remove the chops from the grill and place them on a warmed serving plate. Spoon the marinade over the chops and serve immediately.

# Spiced Liver G W & Y

*Serves 4*

675 g (1½ lb) lamb's liver, thinly sliced
5 cm (2 inch) piece of fresh ginger, peeled and finely grated
4 garlic cloves, crushed
1 teaspoon hot chilli powder
freshly ground black pepper
juice of 1 lemon
1 tablespoon sunflower oil

1. Cut each liver slice in half lengthways. Set aside.

2. Combine the ginger, garlic, chilli powder, pepper and lemon juice in a mixing bowl. Add the liver slices and turn and toss them in the mixture until they are all well coated. Cover the bowl and set aside to marinate for 1 hour.

3. In a large frying pan, heat the oil over a moderate heat. When the oil is very hot add the liver slices, a few at a time, and fry, turning them frequently, for 4–6 minutes or until they are crisp and tender. Using a slotted spoon, remove the liver from the pan and set it aside on a warmed serving dish. Keep hot while you fry the remaining slices in the same way.

# Liver and Sweetcorn W & Y

*Serves 2*

15 ml (1 tablespoon) sunflower oil
50 g (2 oz) onions, chopped
1 small garlic clove, chopped
300 g (10 oz) of liver
100 g (4 oz) can sweetcorn
4 tablespoons (60 ml) vegetable stock
pinch of thyme
black pepper to taste

1. Heat the oil in a frying pan and add the onions and garlic. Sauté for a couple of minutes until the onions are soft.

2. Add the liver and cook, turning occasionally, until browned.

3. Add the sweetcorn and cook for 1 minute longer.

4. Stir in the remaining ingredients and bring to the boil.

5. Reduce the heat, cover and simmer for 2 minutes.

# Liver Kebabs G W & Y

*Serves 4*

675 g (1½ lb) lamb's liver, thickly sliced
15 ml (1 tablespoon) lemon juice (fresh)
freshly ground black pepper to taste
75 ml (3 fl oz) olive oil
4 tablespoons cumin seeds
3 medium onions, thinly sliced

1.  Pre-heat the grill on a moderate heat.

2.  Sprinkle the liver with lemon juice and set aside for 10 minutes. Pat dry with kitchen paper and rub the liver with black pepper. Brush the liver with 30 ml (2 tablespoons) of the oil.

3.  Place the meat on foil and grill for 2 minutes each side. Transfer to a chopping board.

4.  With a sharp knife cut the liver into 5 cm (2 inch) cubes.

5.  Roll the cubes in the cumin seeds. Thread the cubes of liver on to skewers and roll them again in the cumin seeds. Set aside and keep warm.

6.  Heat the remaining olive oil in a frying pan. Add the onions and cook, stirring occasionally, for 5–7 minutes until they are soft.

7.  Place the skewers under the grill and grill the kebabs for 4–6 minutes, turning occasionally, until the liver is tender and cooked through. Serve on a plate and cover with the onions.

# Kidneys in Sesame Sauce G & W

*Serves 2 as a main course, 4 as a starter*

4 pig's kidneys, cleaned and prepared
300 ml (10 fl oz) water
4 tablespoons peanut butter
45 ml (3 tablespoons) vegetable oil
15 ml (1 tablespoon) sesame oil
30 ml (2 tablespoons) soy sauce
45 ml (3 tablespoons) sherry (optional)
2 teaspoons sugar
1 pinch cayenne
2 leeks, white part only, finely chopped

1.  Cut each kidney into 6 slices lengthways.

2.  In a small saucepan bring the water to the boil and drop the kidney slices in. When they change colour remove the pan from the heat and drain the kidneys. Set aside.

3.  In a small bowl mix together the peanut butter, 1 tablespoon of the vegetable oil, the sesame oil, soy sauce, sherry, sugar and cayenne. Set the sauce aside.

4.  In a large frying-pan, heat the remaining vegetable oil over moderate heat. Add the kidneys and leeks and cook them for 4 minutes, stirring constantly.

5.  Using a slotted spoon, remove the kidneys and leeks from the pan. Drain them on kitchen paper and place them on a heated serving dish. Pour the sauce over the kidneys and leeks. Serve immediately.

# 15

# POULTRY

## Chicken and Spinach Stir-fry G & W

*Serves 2*

45 ml (3 tablespoons) vegetable oil
225 g (8 oz) chicken, cut into strips
30 ml (2 tablespoons) soy sauce
15 ml (1 tablespoon) apple juice
freshly ground black pepper to taste
40 g (1½ oz) margarine
450 g (1 lb) spinach, washed, trimmed and chopped

1. Heat the oil and add the chicken strips. Stir-fry for 2 minutes.

2. Add the soy sauce, apple juice and pepper and stir-fry for a further 2 minutes. With a slotted spoon transfer the chicken to a plate.

3. Add 25 g (1 oz) of the margarine to the pan and melt over a moderate heat. Add the spinach and stir-fry for 3 minutes. Add the remaining margarine and fry for a further 30 seconds.

4. Transfer the spinach with a slotted spoon to a warmed serving dish.

5. Increase the heat and return the chicken to the pan. Stir-fry for 30 seconds to reheat thoroughly.

6. Pour the chicken and the pan juices over the spinach and serve immediately.

# Chicken with Peach Sauce G W & Y

## Serves 4

freshly ground black pepper
1.6 kg (3½ lb) fresh chicken, skinned and cut into 6 serving
  pieces
60 ml (2 tablespoons) vegetable oil
1 small onion, finely chopped
1 garlic clove, crushed
¼ teaspoon red pepper flakes
½ teaspoon ground ginger
225 ml (8 fl oz) vegetable stock
50 ml (2 fl oz) lime juice
50 ml (2 fl oz) lemon juice
15 ml (1 tablespoon) sunflower oil
4 fresh peaches, washed, dried, halved, stoned and sliced

1. Pre-heat the oven to 190°C (375°F) gas mark 5.

2. Sprinkle the black pepper over the chicken pieces and set them aside.

3. In a large frying pan heat the oil and add the chicken pieces a few at a time. Fry, turning occasionally, for 8–10 minutes. With a slotted spoon, remove the chicken from the pan and transfer to a medium ovenproof casserole.

4. Add the onion and garlic to the pan and fry them, stirring occasionally, for 5–7 minutes or until the onion is soft and translucent but not brown. Stir in the pepper flakes, ginger and stock and bring the mixture to the boil, stirring constantly.

5. Remove the pan from the heat and stir in the lime and lemon juice. Pour the mixture over the chicken pieces in the casserole. Set aside.

6. Melt the oil in a clean frying pan and gently fry the peaches for 6 minutes, or until they begin to pulp. Transfer from the pan to the casserole.

7. Cover the casserole and bake in pre-heated oven for 1 hour or until the chicken pieces are tender. Serve with rice.

# Grilled Chicken with Herbs G W & Y

## Serves 4

Two 900 g (2 lb) chickens, cut in half lengthways
1 large garlic clove, halved
½ teaspoon freshly ground black pepper
100 g (4 oz) sunflower margarine
30 ml (2 tablespoons) olive oil
juice of ½ lemon
1 tablespoon chopped fresh parsley
1½ teaspoons dried basil

1. Pre-heat the grill to moderate. Rub the chicken halves all over with the garlic cloves and then with the pepper, and set aside.

2. In a small saucepan heat the margarine and oil. Remove from the heat and stir in the lemon juice, parsley and basil.

3. Brush the chicken with the oil and herb mixture, place the chicken halves skin side down on the grill and grill for 7–10 minutes on each side, basting frequently with the oil and herb mixture.

4. After 15 minutes, test the chicken by inserting a skewer into one of the thighs. If the juices run clear, they are cooked.

5. Remove the chicken halves from the grill, transfer to a warmed serving dish and spoon any remaining oil and herb mixture over them.

# Sweet and Sour Chicken G

## Serves 4

350 g (12 oz) chicken breast
pinch of Chinese five spice powder
2 tablespoons flaked almonds
350 g (12 oz) fresh pineapple without skin *or* canned in
    natural juice
50 ml (2 fl oz) wine vinegar
1 tablespoon shoyu soy sauce
1 tablespoon arrowroot
45 ml (3 tablespoons) sunflower oil
4 spring onions, chopped
1 garlic clove, thinly sliced
1 dessertspoon thinly sliced ginger root
1 green pepper, cored, seeded sliced and cut into long strips

1.  Slice the chicken into small, thin slices and sprinkle them with five spice powder.

2.  Toast the almonds under the grill until they are lightly browned.

3.  Blend 100 g (4 oz) of the pineapple with the wine vinegar, soy sauce and arrowroot. Cut the remaining pineapple into 2.5 cm (1 inch) chunks and reserve.

4.  Heat 1 tablespoon of the oil in a wok or frying pan and stir in the onions, garlic and ginger. Fry for 1 minute and remove to a plate.

5.  Heat the rest of the oil in the pan and toss the chicken slices in it until just browned, 3–5 minutes.

6.  Add the pepper and stir for about 1 minute. Add the cooked onion, garlic and ginger, pineapple chunks and toasted almond flakes.

7.  Pour the pineapple and vinegar liquid over the top and stir for a few minutes. Serve immediately.

# Hot Fruity Chicken G

## Serves 2

15 ml (1 tablespoon) concentrated apple juice
1 garlic clove, chopped
2 teaspoons peeled, grated ginger
10 ml (2 teaspoons) chilli sauce
300 g (10 oz) chicken breast, skinned and boned, and cut into
    thin strips
10 ml (2 teaspoons) sunflower oil
150 g (5 oz) onions, sliced
1 medium green pepper, cored, seeded and chopped
1 teaspoon cornflour
black pepper
2 large oranges, peeled, segmented and pith removed

1. Mix together the apple juice, half the garlic, the ginger and the chilli sauce. Add the chicken and coat throughly.

2. Cover and refrigerate for at least 1 hour to marinate. It can be left overnight.

3. Remove the chicken and reserve the marinade.

4. Heat the oil and sauté the onions and remaining garlic until the onions are transparent.

5. Add the chicken and chopped pepper and cook until the chicken is lightly browned on both sides.

6. Strain the reserved marinade and mix it with the cornflower.

7. Add the cornflour mixture and black pepper to taste to the pan. Bring to the boil, stirring constantly. Reduce the heat to a simmer.

8. Add the orange segments and heat through thoroughly, stirring occasionally. Serve immediately.

# Chicken with Almonds G & W

## Serves 4 to 6

1 x 5 lb chicken, cut into 8 serving pieces
30 ml (2 tablespoons) vegetable oil
1 large onion, finely chopped
2 garlic cloves, crushed (optional)
1 large green pepper, seeded and chopped
1 large red pepper, seeded and chopped
425 ml (15 fl oz) chicken stock
1 pinch of cayenne pepper
bouquet garni, consisting of 4 parsley sprigs, 1 thyme spray
    and 1 bay leaf tied together
2 hard-boiled egg yolks
50 g (2 oz) ground almonds

1.  Heat the oil in a large flameproof casserole over a moderate heat. Add the chicken and brown gently on both sides.

2.  Remove the chicken and set aside.

3.  Add the onion, garlic and green pepper. Stir occasionally for 5 to 7 minutes or until the onion is soft but not brown.

4.  Add the chicken to the casserole with the stock, cayenne and bouquet garni. Bring the liquid to the boil, reduce heat and simmer for 40 minutes or until the chicken pieces are tender.

5.  In a small bowl mash the egg yolks and 3 tablespoons of the cooking liquid together with a fork until the mixture forms a smooth paste. Add the ground almonds and combine the mixture thoroughly.

6.  Stir the paste into the casserole a little at a time, simmer for a further 10 minutes.

7.  Remove the chicken pieces from the casserole and transfer to a warmed serving dish. Discard the bouquet garni, and continue

to boil the sauce stirring occasionally for 3 to 5 minutes until it has thickened slightly.

8.   Remove the casserole from the heat and pour the sauce over the chicken. Serve immediately.

# Chicken with Grapes and Peanuts G & W

## Serves 6–8

30 ml (2 tablespoons) groundnut oil
900 g (2 lb) chicken breasts, cut into 2.5 cm (1 inch) cubes
freshly ground black pepper to taste
65 g (2½ oz) unsalted peanuts, ground
30 ml (2 tablespoons) soy sauce
good pinch of mild chilli powder
450 g (1 lb) seedless white grapes, halved
75 g (3 oz) unsalted peanuts, finely chopped and toasted

1.   Heat the oil over a moderate heat. Add the chicken and cook for 5 minutes, or until the cubes are browned.

2.   Add the pepper, ground peanuts, soy sauce and chilli powder and mix well.

3.   Reduce the heat and add the grapes. Simmer for 15–20 minutes, until the chicken is tender.

4.   Remove from the heat and transfer to a warmed serving dish. Sprinkle with the chopped peanuts and serve.

# Turkey Breast with Mushroom Sauce W

*Serves 4*

2 tablespoons of vegetable oil
1 medium-sized onion, finely chopped
1 garlic clove, crushed (optional)
4 turkey breasts
25 g (1 oz) margarine
400 g (14 oz) mushrooms, wiped clean and sliced
450 ml (16 fl oz) chicken stock
1 teaspoon chopped fresh thyme or ½ teaspoon dried thyme
black pepper to taste
1 bay leaf
2 tablespoons cornflour dissolved in 6 tablespoons water

1. Heat the oil in a frying pan and add the onion, garlic and turkey breasts. Cook turning frequently for 8 to 10 minutes until evenly brown.

2. Remove the onion, garlic and turkey and set aside. Drain off the oil and add the margarine to the pan with the mushrooms. Stir constantly for 3 minutes. Remove from pan and set aside.

3. In a large frameproof casserole, heat the stock, thyme, pepper and bay leaf. Stir in the cornflour mixture. Stir constantly until the mixture begins to thicken.

4. Add the turkey, onion, garlic and mushrooms to the casserole, stir well.

5. Reduce heat to low, cover and simmer for 20 to 25 minutes or until the turkey is tender. Remove bay leaf and serve.

# Turkey and Chickpeas with Rice G W & Y

*Serves 4*

50 g (2 oz) margarine
12 pickling onions
900 g (2 lb) turkey breast, cut into 2.5 cm (1 inch) cubes
100 g (4 oz) chickpeas, soaked overnight and drained
225 ml (8 fl oz) vegetable stock
freshly ground black pepper
1 teaspoon ground cumin
pinch of turmeric
450 g (1 lb) long-grain rice, washed, soaked in cold water for
    30 minutes and drained

1.  Melt the margarine in a large pan over a moderate heat. Add the onions and turkey cubes and cook, stirring and turning, for 5–8 minutes, until the onions are golden.

2.  Add the chickpeas, stock and add enough water to cover the mixture completely.

3.  Add the pepper to taste, cumin and turmeric to the pan and stir well to blend. Cover the pan and cook for 1¼ hours or until the turkey and chickpeas are tender.

4.  Raise the heat and bring the liquid to the boil. Stir in the rice. Cover the pan, reduce the heat and simmer for 15–20 minutes or until the rice is tender and the liquid absorbed.

5.  Remove the pan from the heat, spoon the mixture into a warmed serving dish and serve immediately.

# Parsley and Lemon Stuffing G W & Y

*Enough to stuff a 4–4.5 kg (9–10 lb) chicken or turkey*

300 g (10 oz) cooked brown rice
grated rind *and* juice of 2 lemons
4 tablespoons chopped fresh parsley
¼ teaspoon dried thyme
1 teaspoon grated orange rind
¼ teaspoon dried marjoram
50 g (2 oz) margarine
75 ml (3 fl oz) orange juice
1 egg (size 3) beaten

1. In a medium mixing bowl combine the rice, lemon rind, parsley, orange rind, thyme, marjoram and margarine.

2. Stir in the orange juice, lemon juice and egg and blend well.

3. Stuff the chicken or turkey in the usual way.

# 16

# EGG AND VEGETARIAN DISHES AND SAVOURY SAUCES

## Spanish Rice G & W

*Serves 3–4*

45 ml (3 tablespoons) olive oil
2 onions, thinly sliced
2 garlic cloves, crushed
1 green pepper, cored, seeded and thinly sliced
2 red peppers, cored, seeded and thinly sliced
350 g (12 oz) mushrooms, thinly sliced
400 g (14 oz) canned, chopped tomatoes
40 g (1½ oz) stoned green olives (optional)
1 teaspoon dried oregano
½ teaspoon basil
freshly ground black pepper to taste
150 g (5 oz) cooked rice

1. Heat the oil in a large frying pan. Add the onions and garlic and cook for 5–7 minutes, stirring occasionally.

2. Add the green and red peppers and cook for 4 minutes, stirring frequently. Add the mushrooms, tomatoes with their juice, olives, oregano, basil and pepper to the pan and cook, stirring occasionally, for 3 minutes.

3. Add the rice to the pan and cook for 3–4 minutes, stirring constantly until the rice is heated through.

4. Serve immediately, if serving hot.

# Nut Croquettes W & Y

*Serves 4*

25 g (1 oz) sunflower margarine
1 small onion, finely chopped
25 g (1 oz) flour *plus* 30 ml (2 tablespoons)
150 ml (5 fl oz) milk
100 g (4 oz) unsalted peanuts, finely chopped
1 small carrot, peeled and finely grated
¼ teaspoon dried thyme
¼ teaspoon freshly ground black pepper
4 tablespoons sunflower oil

1.  Melt the margarine in a saucepan, add the onions and cook until soft.

2.  Stir in 25 g (1 oz) of the flour to make a smooth paste.

3.  Remove the pan from the heat and, stirring constantly, gradually add the milk. Return to the heat and, stirring constantly, bring to the boil. Boil for 1 minute until very thick.

4.  Remove the pan from the heat and add the peanuts, carrot, thyme and pepper and mix thoroughly.

5.  Spoon into a medium dish and set aside to cool.

6.  Cut the mixture into 5.25 cm (2×1 inch) pieces and roll them in the remaining flour.

7.  In a large frying pan heat the oil. When hot, add half the croquettes and fry for 4 minutes until golden brown. Remove from the frying pan with a slotted spoon on to kitchen paper. Keep them warm while you cook the remaining croquettes.

# Spiced Lentil Cakes W & Y

## Serves 5

225 g (8 oz) green lentils
vegetable oil for frying
1 garlic clove, crushed
2 carrots, peeled and chopped
1 small onion, chopped
2 teaspoons ground cumin
2 teaspoons ground coriander
finely grated rind and juice of ½ orange
3 tablespoons fresh chopped parsley
50 g (2 oz) fresh, white breadcrumbs
freshly ground black pepper
2 eggs, size 3, beaten
50 g (2 oz) dry white breadcrumbs, sieved
parsley
wedges of lemon

1.  Cook the lentils in boiling water for 30–35 minutes. Drain and refresh under cold water. Drain thoroughly again.

2.  Meanwhile, heat 30 ml (2 tablespoons) vegetable oil in a pan. Add the garlic, carrots and onion. Cover and cook gently, shaking the pan occasionally, for 15 minutes. Cool.

3.  Place the lentils and vegetables in a blender or food processor with the coriander, cumin, orange rind and juice and blend until smooth. Transfer to a bowl, stir in the parsley and fresh breadcrumbs, and season with black pepper.

4.  Divide the mixture into 10 portions and form into flat cakes, pressing firmly to remove any cracks. Dip the cakes into the beaten egg and then in the dry breadcrumbs. Chill for 30 minutes.

5.  Heat 6 mm (¼ inch) vegetable oil in a frying pan and fry the lentil cakes for 3–4 minutes on each side until golden brown. Garnish with parsley and lemon wedges.

# Vegetable and Dal Jackets W

*Serves 4*

30 ml (2 tablespoons) vegetable oil
1 small onion, chopped
1 tablespoon mild curry powder
75 g (3 oz) red lentils
75 g (3 oz) French beans, trimmed and cut into 2.5 cm
   (1 inch) lengths
50 g (2 oz) raisins
25 g (1 oz) desiccated coconut
200 ml (7 fl oz) vegetable stock
400 g (14 oz) canned, chopped tomatoes
4 hot baked potatoes
freshly ground black pepper
toasted, flaked coconut to garnish

1. Heat the oil and sauté the onion for 3 minutes, until soft.

2. Add the curry powder and lentils and cook for 5 minutes, stirring occasionally.

3. Add the beans, raisins, coconut, stock and tomatoes, cover and simmer for 20 minutes, stirring frequently.

4. Cut the tops off the potatoes and scoop out the centres. Cut the potato into chunks, add to the vegetable dal and season with black pepper.

5. Spoon a little of the vegetable mixture into the potato skins and serve the remainder separately.

6. Garnish with a little toasted coconut.

# Chickpea Dip W & Y

## Serves 8

Two 850 g (15 oz) cans chickpeas, drained and rinsed
1 garlic clove, crushed
15 ml (1 tablespoon) lemon juice (fresh)
25 ml (1 fl oz) olive oil
175 ml (6 fl oz) Greek plain yogurt
freshly ground black pepper
4 teaspoons freshly chopped parsley
10 ml (2 teaspoons) tomato purée
sprigs of parsley *and* strips of red pepper *and* pieces of sliced
    lemon to garnish
selection of raw vegetables – peppers, radishes, carrots, celery,
    cucumber – to serve

1.  Place the chickpeas in a blender or food processor and blend until smooth.

2.  Add the garlic, lemon juice, olive oil and yogurt and mix well. Add black pepper to taste.

3.  Transfer one-third of the mixture to a small serving bowl. Divide the rest between 2 small mixing bowls.

4.  Add the chopped parsley to one, stir well and transfer to a small serving bowl.

5.  Add the tomato puree to the other, stir well and transfer to a small serving bowl. Adjust seasoning if necessary.

6.  Garnish the herb dip with sprigs of parsley, the tomato dip with red pepper and the plain dip with pieces of lemon.

7.  Chop the vegetables into sticks. Arrange on a serving dish around the dips.

# Egg and Vegetable Bake G W & Y

*Serves 6*

15 ml (1 tablespoon) olive oil
2 garlic cloves, crushed
2 medium onions, finely chopped
6 large tomatoes, peeled and finely chopped
1 green chilli, seeded and finely chopped
5 ml (1 teaspoon) apple juice
freshly ground black pepper
½ teaspoon ground coriander
12 eggs
175 g (6 oz) Cheddar cheese, grated
1 tablespoon margarine
pinch of chilli powder

1.  Pre-heat the oven to 230°C (450°F) gas mark 8.

2.  Heat the oil in a large frying pan. Add the onions and garlic and fry for 5–7 minutes, stirring occasionally.

3.  Add the tomatoes, chilli, apple juice, pepper and coriander to the pan. Reduce the heat and simmer the mixture, stirring frequently, for 15–20 minutes or until it is soft and pulpy.

4.  Transfer the mixture to a large ovenproof dish.

5.  With the back of a spoon, make 12 hollows in the mixture. Place one egg in each hollow.

6.  Sprinkle the cheese over the eggs. Dot the margarine over the cheese and sprinkle the chilli powder over the top.

7.  Bake in the centre of the oven for 6–8 minutes or until the cheese is golden brown and the eggs have set.

8.  Serve immediately.

# Courgette and Tomato Quiche W & Y

## Serves 4–6

250 g (8 oz) shortcrust pastry
50 g (2 oz) margarine
2 garlic cloves, crushed
4 courgettes, trimmed and sliced
freshly ground black pepper to taste
½ teaspoon oregano
100 ml (4 fl oz) milk
3 eggs
50 g (2 oz) Cheddar cheese, grated
5 small tomatoes, peeled and thinly sliced

1. Line a flan dish with the pastry and set aside.

2. Pre-heat the oven to 200°C (400°F) gas mark 6.

3. Melt the margarine in a large frying pan.

4. Add the garlic and fry, stirring frequently, for 1 minute.

5. Add the courgettes and pepper. Fry for 8–10 minutes or until lightly browned.

6. Remove the pan from the heat and add the oregano, mixing well to blend.

7. In a mixing bowl combine the milk, eggs and cheese. Beat well to blend.

8. Arrange the courgettes and tomatoes in circles in the pastry flan case.

9. Pour the egg, milk and cheese mixture over the courgettes and tomatoes.

10. Place in the centre of the oven and bake for 35–45 minutes or until the filling is set and golden brown.

# Potato and Cheese Bake W & Y

## Serves 4

700 g (1½ lb) potatoes, peeled
50 g (2 oz) margarine
2 medium onions, finely chopped
25 g (1 oz) flour
freshly ground black pepper to taste
½ teaspoon dried mixed herbs
350 ml (12 fl oz) milk
225 g (8 oz) Cheddar cheese, finely grated

1.  Pre-heat the oven to 180°C (350°F) gas mark 4.

2.  Boil and mash the potatoes. Place them in a medium mixing bowl and set aside.

3.  With a teaspoon of margarine, grease a medium ovenproof dish.

4.  Melt the remaining margarine in a saucepan over a moderate heat. Add the onions and fry until softened and golden.

5.  Remove the pan from the heat and with a wooden spoon stir in the flour, black pepper and herbs to make a smooth paste.

6.  Gradually add the milk, stirring constantly and being careful to avoid lumps.

7.  Return the pan to a low heat, stirring constantly, for 4–5 minutes or until the sauce is smooth and thick.

8.  Add 175g (6 oz) of the cheese and cook until it has melted, stirring all the time.

9.  Gradually pour the cheese sauce over the potatoes, beating constantly with a wooden spoon until the mixture is smooth.

10. Turn the mixture into the prepared dish and smooth the mixtue down with the back of a spoon. Sprinkle with the remaining cheese.

11. Place the dish in the centre of the oven and bake for 20–25 minutes or until the top is golden brown.

12. Serve immediately.

# Mexican Stuffed Eggs G & W

*Serves 6*

6 hard-boiled eggs
1 medium avocado, peeled, stoned and chopped
1 small onion, finely minced
1 small green pepper, cored, seeded and finely minced
100 g (4 oz) prawns *or* shrimps, shelled, deveined and finely
  chopped
5 ml (1 teaspoon) lemon juice
5 ml (1 teaspoon) wine vinegar
freshly ground black pepper to taste
1 pinch of cayenne pepper
15 ml (1 tablespoon) chopped freshly parsley

1. Slice the eggs in half lengthways and scoop out the yolks. Set the whites aside. Using the back of a wooden spoon rub the yolks and the avocado flesh through a fine nylon strainer into a medium mixing bowl. Stir in the onion, green pepper and chopped prawns.

2. Add the lemon juice, vinegar, pepper and cayenne, mixing well to blend.

3. With a teaspoon, generously stuff the egg white halves with the mixture. Arrange on a serving dish, sprinkle with parsley and chill before serving.

# Nut and Vegetable Loaf G W & Y

*Serves 4–6*

10 ml (2 teaspoons) sunflower oil
1 small onion, chopped
1 small carrot, chopped
1 stick celery, chopped
15 ml (1 tablespoon) tomato purée
225 g (8 oz) tomatoes, skinned and chopped
2 eggs
1 tablespoon chopped parsley
freshly ground black pepper
225 g (8 oz) nuts, finely chopped or minced
onion rings
parsley sprigs

1. Pre-heat the oven to 220°C (425°F) gas mark 7.

2. Melt the oil in a pan, add the onion, carrot and celery and cook until softened. Add the tomato puree and tomatoes and cook for 5 minutes.

3. Put the eggs, parsley and pepper to taste in a bowl and beat well. Stir in the nuts and vegetables.

4. Transfer to a greased 900 ml (1½ pint) ovenproof dish and bake for 30–35 minutes.

5. Turn out and decorate with onion rings and parsley. Serve hot with vegetables and sauce, or cold with salad.

# Peanut Savoury Pie G & W

*Serves 4*

30 ml (2 tablespoons) groundnut oil
1 large onion, sliced
335 g (8 oz) roasted peanuts, chopped
226 g (8 oz) can tomatoes
5 ml (1 teaspoon) Worcestershire sauce
1 teaspoon chopped mixed herbs
freshly ground black pepper
225 g (8 oz) shortcrust pastry
1 egg, beaten

1. Pre-heat the oven to 200°C (400°F) gas mark 6.

2. Heat the oil in a frying pan, add the onion and fry for about 10 minutes until softened. Stir in the nuts, tomatoes with their juice, Worcestershire sauce, herbs and pepper to taste. Bring to the boil and simmer for 2–3 minutes. Remove from the heat and leave to cool.

3. Divide the prepared pastry in half. Roll out one piece on a floured surface and use to line a 20 cm (8 inch) pie plate. Spoon in the filling. Roll out the remaining pastry and cover the pie. Glaze with beaten egg. Knock up the edges, seal well and flute.

4. Bake for 35–40 minutes, until golden. Serve hot or cold, with vegetables of your choice or salad.

# Bean and Tomato Hot-Pot G & W

*Serves 4*

30 ml (2 tablespoons) sunflower oil
2 onions, sliced
3 carrots, sliced
2 sticks celery, sliced
1 large leek, sliced
2 garlic cloves, crushed
425 g (15 oz) can red kidney beans, drained
396 g (14 oz) can tomatoes
300 ml (½ pint) stock
1 tablespoon yeast extract
freshly ground black pepper
750 g (1½ lb) potatoes, thinly sliced
15 g (½ oz) margarine

1.  Pre-heat the oven to 180°C (350°F) gas mark 4.

2.  Heat the oil in a flameproof casserole, add the onions and fry for 5 minutes. Add the carrots, celery, leek and garlic and fry for a further 5 minutes.

3.  Add the kidney beans, tomatoes with their juice, stock, yeast extract, and pepper to taste. Mix well.

4.  Arrange the potatoes neatly on top, sprinkling pepper between each layer. Dot with the margarine, cover and cook in the oven for 2 hours.

5.  Remove the lid 30 minutes before the end of cooking to allow the potatoes to brown.

# Bean and Egg Au Gratin Y

*Serves 4*

450 g (1 lb) shelled broad beans
3 hard-boiled eggs, sliced
50 g (2 oz) margarine
40 g (1½ oz) wholewheat flour
450 ml (¾ pint) milk
freshly ground black pepper
2 tablespoons fresh brown breadcrumbs
50 g (2 oz) Cheddar cheese, grated

1.  Pre-heat the oven to 220°C (425°F) gas mark 7.

2.  Cook the beans in boiling water until just tender, and drain. Put half the beans in a greased ovenproof dish, place the eggs on top and cover with the remaining beans.

3.  Melt 40 g (14 oz) of the margarine in a pan, stir in the flour and cook gently, stirring. Remove from the heat and gradually add the milk, stirring continuously. Return to the heat and bring to the boil. Cook, stirring, until thickened. Season to taste with pepper.

4.  Pour the sauce over the beans and sprinkle the breadcrumbs and cheese over the top. Dot with the remaining margarine and bake for 15 minutes, until golden brown. Serve immediately.

# Oaty Cheese Quiche W

*Serves 4–6*

*Pastry*
75 g (3 oz) self-raising flour
150 g (5 oz) fine oatmeal
freshly ground black pepper
100 g (4 oz) vegetable margarine
dried beans for baking 'blind'

*Filling*
350 g (12 oz) cottage cheese, sieved
30 ml (2 tablespoons) natural yogurt
6 sticks celery, chopped
75 g (3 oz) hazelnuts, chopped
pinch of curry powder

*Garnish*
pinch of paprika
tomato slices
parsley sprigs

1. Pre-heat the oven to 200°C (400°F) gas mark 6.

2. Mix the flour and oatmeal together, with freshly ground pepper to taste. Cut in the margarine and rub in until the mixture resembles breadcrumbs. Stir in enough water to make a fairly stiff pastry and knead together lightly.

3. Turn on to a floured surface, roll out and use to line a 23 cm (9 inch) flan ring. Cover the base with greaseproof paper and fill with dried beans. Bake 'blind' for 20 minutes. Remove the paper and beans and return the flan to the oven for 5 minutes. Allow to cool.

4. Mix the cheese, yogurt, celery, nuts and curry powder together and pile into the flan case. Sprinkle with paprika and garnish with tomato and parsley.

# Corn and Asparagus Flan Y

## *Serves 4–6*

225 g (8 oz) wholewheat pastry
198 g (7 oz) can sweetcorn, drained
141 g (5 oz) can asparagus tips, drained
1 small onion, chopped
75 g (3 oz) Cheddar cheese, grated
2 large eggs, beaten
300 ml (½ pint) milk
freshly ground black pepper

1.  Pre-heat the oven to 200°C (400°F) gas mark 6.

2.  Roll out the prepared pastry and line a 20 cm (8 inch) flan tin. Cover the base with greaseproof paper and fill with dried beans. Bake 'blind' for 10 minutes. Remove the paper and beans and bake for a further 15 minutes.

3.  Mix the sweetcorn, asparagus, onion, cheese, eggs and milk together. Add pepper to taste and pour into the prepared flan case.

4.  Lower the oven temperature to 190°C (375°F) gas mark 5 and return the flan to the oven for 30 minutes until set. Serve hot or cold.

# Potato and Herb Omelette W & Y

*Serves 4*

450 g (1 lb) potatoes, cooked and mashed
3 eggs, separated
30 ml (2 tablespoons) milk
1 tablespoon mixed herbs
freshly ground black pepper
10 ml (2 teaspoons) sunflower oil
cucumber *and* tomato slices

1.  Beat the potato with the egg yolks, milk, mixed herbs and pepper to taste.

2.  Whisk the egg whites until stiff and fold them into the potato mixture.

3.  Melt the butter in an omelette pan, add the mixture and cook for 2 minutes on each side.

4.  Slide on to a serving plate and cut into quarters. Garnish each portion with cucumber and tomato. Serve with green salad or vegetables.

# Spinach and Tomato Omelette G W & Y

*Serves 1*

2 eggs (size 3)
freshly ground black pepper
50 g (2 oz) fresh spinach (cooked in a little boiling water for
    3–4 minutes, and drained
2 medium tomatoes, sliced

1.  Beat the eggs and mix with pepper to taste.

2.  Pour into a hot frying pan and leave to set for ½ minute.

3.  Add the spinach and tomato and leave for about a minute until heated through.

4.  Fold in half and serve.

# Baked Nutty Onions G W & Y

*Serves 4*

300 g (10 oz) onions, peeled and sliced
1 bay leaf
300 ml (½ pint) skimmed milk
25 g (1 oz) sunflower margarine
25 g (1 oz) flour
freshly ground black pepper
1 teaspoon ground nutmeg
150 g (5 oz) unsalted peanuts, finely chopped
2 tomatoes, halved and grilled

1.  Pre-heat the oven to 190°C (375°F) gas mark 5.

2.  Place the onion, bay leaf and milk in a saucepan and bring to the boil. Cover, and simmer for 10 minutes.

3.  Strain the milk into a jug, discard the bay leaf and place the onions in a greased ovenproof dish.

4.  Melt the margarine in a small pan. When foaming, stir in the flour and cook for 1 minute. Gradually add the milk, stirring continuously. Cook until thick and smooth. Add pepper and nutmeg to taste.

5.  Pour the sauce over the onions and sprinkle evenly with nuts. Bake for 20–30 minutes. Reduce the heat if the nuts are browning too quickly. Garnish with the tomatoes.

# Nutty Sprout Stir-fry G & W

## Serves 2–4

75 g (3 oz) unsalted peanuts
1 medium orange, peeled and cut into segments
10 ml (2 teaspoons) oil
1 pinch of cayenne
½ teaspoon ground cumin
2 thick spring onions, trimmed and sliced
1 garlic clove, thinly sliced
175 g (6 oz) Brussels sprouts, trimmed and thinly sliced
1 red pepper, cored, seeded and thinly sliced
2 tablespoons (30 ml) soy sauce (avoid for low-yeast diet)

1.  Place the peanuts on a baking dish in a pre-heated oven (180°C/375°F, gas mark 5) until they are lightly roasted.

2.  Slice the orange segments crossways into triangles.

3.  Heat the oil in a wok or heavy frying pan. Add the cayenne, cumin, spring onions, garlic and sprouts and toss in the oil for 1 minute.

4.  Add the roasted peanuts and red pepper, mix and fry again for 1 minute.

5.  Lastly add the orange triangles and soy sauce and stir-fry until all the vegetables are coated and the oranges are heated through. Serve immediately.

# Spinach Gratin W & Y

*Serves 4*

2 slices dry wholewheat bread (or white if on a wholewheat-
  restricted diet)
50 g (2 oz) Gruyère cheese
450 g (1 lb) fresh *or* frozen spinach, cooked and drained well
½ teaspoon grated nutmeg
freshly ground black pepper

1.  Pre-heat the oven to 230°C (450°F) gas mark 8.

2.  Break up the bread into rough breadcrumbs.

3.  Grate the cheese.

4.  Mix the spinach with the nutmeg, pepper to taste and half the
    grated cheese, and place in an ovenproof dish.

5.  Mix the remaining cheese with the breadcrumbs and sprinkle
    them over the top.

6.  Bake for about 15 minutes until golden brown.

# Vegetable Curry G & W

*Serves 2*

2 teaspoons vegetable oil
1 garlic clove, crushed
¼ teaspoon turmeric
¼ teaspoon coriander
¼ teaspoon cumin seeds
1 teaspoon finely chopped ginger
½ small chilli, seeded and finely chopped
2 tablespoons tomato purée
850 ml (1½ pints) vegetable stock
175 g (6 oz) boiled butter beans
75 g (3 oz) cauliflower, broken into florets
75 g (3 oz) turnip, cut into 2.5 cm (1 inch) cubes

75 g (3 oz) parsnip, cut into 2.5 cm (1 inch) cubes
75 g (3 oz) courgettes, thickly sliced
1 small onion, chopped

1. Heat the oil in a saucepan. Add the garlic, spices and chilli, and stir over a moderate heat for 1 minute.

2. Add all the remaining ingredients, mix well and bring to the boil.

3. Cover and simmer for 15 minutes, then for a further 10 minutes without a lid.

4. Serve with brown rice and salad.

# Mustard Sauce G & W

*Makes about 300 ml (10 fl oz)*

1 tablespoon margarine
1 garlic clove, crushed
1½ tablespoons flour
freshly ground black pepper to taste
300 ml (10 fl oz) milk
1 tablespoon prepared French *or* German mustard
5 ml (1 teaspoon) lemon juice

1. Melt the margarine in a saucepan over a moderate heat. Add the garlic and cook for 4 minutes.

2. Remove the pan from the heat and stir in the flour with a wooden spoon. Add the pepper and make into a smooth paste. Gradually stir in the milk, avoiding the sauce turning lumpy.

3. Stir in the mustard thoroughly.

4. Cook the sauce over a low heat for 3–4 minutes until it has thickened. Do not let the sauce boil.

5. Remove the pan from the heat and stir in the lemon juice. Pour into a sauce boat and serve immediately.

# Orange and Herb Sauce W & Y

*Serves 4*

10 ml (2 teaspoons) sunflower oil
1 small onion, finely chopped
175 ml (6 fl oz) frozen concentrated orange juice
2 teaspoons chopped tarragon
2 teaspoons chopped parsley
black pepper
2 teaspoons cornflour
1 orange, peeled, segmented, pith removed and chopped

1. Heat the oil and gently fry the onions. Add the orange juice, herbs and black pepper to taste.

2. Bring to the boil and simmer for 2–3 minutes.

3. Mix the cornflour with 1 tablespoon cold water and stir into the sauce, bringing slowly to the boil and stirring constantly.

4. Add the chopped orange segments, heat for 1–2 minutes and serve.

This sauce can be used to complement meat and fish dishes as well as vegetarian ones, and can be made in larger quantities in advance and frozen.

# 17

# SWEETS AND CAKES

## Dried Fruit Compote G & W

*Serves 2*

100 g (4 oz) mixture of dried fruits, e.g. peaches, prunes,
    apples, apricots and pears
75 ml (5 level tablespoons) orange juice
2 whole cloves
Two 2.5 cm (1 inch) sticks cinnamon
zest *and* juice of ½ lemon

1.    Wash the fruit and place it in a bowl with the orange juice, spices, lemon juice and zest.

2.    Leave to soak overnight.

3.    Next day, if the juice has been absorbed add 2 tablespoons water. Then place the mixture in a saucepan, bring to the boil, cover and simmer on a very low heat for 10–15 minutes.

4.    Transfer to a serving bowl, removing the cinnamon and cloves. Leave to cool or serve warm.

# Rhubarb and Ginger Mousse G & W

*Serves 4*

450 g (1 lb) rhubarb
3 tablespoons clear honey
juice and grated rind of ½ orange
¼ teaspoon ground ginger
30 ml (2 tablespoons) water
2 teaspoons powdered gelatine
2 egg whites

1. Trim the rhubarb and chop into 2.5cm (1 inch) pieces.

2. Put the rhubarb into a pan with the honey, orange juice, rind and the ginger, and simmer gently until the fruit is soft.

3. Dissolve the gelatine in 2 tablespoons of water, placing the bowl in hot water. Stir until the gelatine is dissolved.

4. Add the gelatine mixture to the fruit and beat until smooth.

5. Cool the rhubarb mixture until it is half-set.

6. Whisk the egg whites until stiff and fold them lightly into the half-set rhubarb mixture.

7. Spoon into decorative glasses and chill until set.

# Baked Apple G W & Y

*Serves 1*

1 cooking apple
1 dessertspoon concentrated apple juice
1 cup water
1 pinch of cinnamon

1. Pre-heat the oven to 180°C (350°F) for gas mark 4.

2. Wash and core the apple, and score around the centre in a circle, just breaking the skin.

3. Place the apple in an ovenproof dish.

4. Mix the apple juice with the cinnamon.

5. Pour the water into the dish, and pour the apple juice over the apple.

6. Bake for approximately 50–60 minutes.

# Melon Ice Cream G W & Y

*Serves 4*

1 medium melon (ogen or similar if you can get it)
285 ml (½ pint) plain yogurt
concentrated apple juice to sweeten if necessary
melon balls to decorate

1. Halve the melon, scoop out the seeds, then scoop out the melon flesh and place it in the blender or food processor.

2. Liquidize the melon flesh and mix with the yogurt and concentrated apple juice as needed.

3. Place the melon and yogurt mixture in a shallow dish and freeze until firm.

4. Scoop the melon ice cream into dessert glasses and decorate with melon balls.

# Orange Jelly G W & Y

*Serves 8*

4 large oranges
2 teaspoons agar powder
100 ml (4 oz) apple juice

1.  Cut the oranges in half and scoop out the flesh.

2.  Put the empty orange halves to one side.

3.  Remove the pith and pips from the orange segments and blend the flesh in a blender or food processor.

4.  Mix the agar powder with a little of the apple juice. Pour this into a saucepan with the rest of the apple juice and a little of the blended orange.

5.  Bring to the boil and cook gently for 1½ minutes.

6.  Take the pan off the heat and add the mixture to the rest of the blended oranges. Mix well.

7.  Leave the mixture to cool slightly, then pour it into the 8 orange halves.

# Apple Custard G W & Y

*Serves 4*

450 g (1 lb) eating apples, sliced
150 ml (5 oz) water
½ teaspoon ground cinnamon
2 eggs

1.  Pre-heat the oven to 180°C (350°F) gas mark 4.

2.  Place the apples, water and cinnamon in a saucepan and cook gently until the apple softens and most of the water is absorbed.

3.  Blend in a blender or food processor and allow to cool for 5–10 minutes.

4.  Whisk the eggs and add a little at a time to the apple purée.

5.  Pour the custard into a 20 cm (8 in) baking dish and bake for 25–30 minutes until browned on top and firm. Serve immediately.

# Apple and Passion Fruit Delight G W & Y

*Serves 4*

4 large eating apples (about 800 g/1¾ lb), chopped
¼ cup water
3 medium passion fruits
1 tablespoon concentrated apple juice
1 teaspoon grated orange rind
3 egg whites

1.  Place the apples and water in a saucepan and bring to the boil. Cover, reduce the heat and simmer for 5 minutes or until the apples are tender.

2.  Add the passion fruits, apple juice and orange rind and stir well, then leave to cool.

3.  Beat the egg whites in a bowl until soft peaks form. Fold this into apple mixture, and refrigerate for 1 hour before serving.

# Fruit Mousse G W & Y

*Serves 4*

100 ml (4 fl oz) apricot nectar
100 ml (4 fl oz) pear juice
2 teaspoons gelatine
30 ml (2 tablespoons) water
2 teaspoons sugar
1 egg, separated
1 medium fresh peach

1.  Mix the two juices and pour into a bowl.

2.  Sprinkle the gelatine over the water, dissolve over hot water and allow to cool to room temperature.

3.  Mix the sugar, egg yolk and gelatine mixture in a bowl, then add to the bowl containing the fruit juice, and refrigerate until slightly thick.

4.  Beat the egg white in a small bowl until soft peaks form. Add to the fruit mixture and fold in lightly.

5.  Refrigerate until set and decorate with fresh fruit.

# Fresh Fruit Salad G W & Y

*Serves 4*

1 dessert apple, peeled and sliced
1 banana, peeled and sliced
4 tablespoons lemon juice
1 orange, peeled and segmented
1 grapefruit, peeled and segmented
100 g (4 oz) seedless grapes
2 kiwi fruit, peeled and sliced
2 tablespoons orange juice
4 sprigs mint

1.  Toss the apple and banana in the lemon juice. This will prevent discoloration.

2.  Combine all the fruits in a serving bowl. Serve chilled and decorate with a sprig of mint.

# Baked Bananas G W & Y

*Serves 6*

6 large bananas unpeeled
1 tablespoon vegetable oil

1.  Pre-heat the oven to 170°C (325°F) gas mark 3.

2.  Rub the banana skins with the vegetable oil. Brush an oven-proof dish with the remaining oil.

3.  Lay the bananas in the dish and place in the centre of the oven.

4.  Bake for 30–40 minutes or until they are soft and the skins have turned black.

5.  Serve hot with one strip of the skin peeled back.

# Banana and Tofu Cream G & W

*Serves 4*

200 g (7 oz) firm tofu
200 g (7 oz) bananas, skinned
75 g (3 oz) ground almonds
1 pinch of cinnamon
2 teaspoons almond flakes

1. Blend or process the tofu and bananas together. To obtain a creamy texture, the mixture may need to be put through a sieve or food mill.

2. Add the ground almonds and mix well.

3. Spoon into 4 bowls or glasses and sprinkle lightly with the cinnamon and a few almond flakes.

# Nutty Carob Slice G & W

*Makes 8 slices*

50 g (2 oz) raisins, chopped and soaked in 25 ml (1½ tablespoons) water for 20 minutes
100 g (4 oz) smooth peanut butter (sugar- and salt-free)
25 g (1 oz) carob powder
50 g (2 oz) sesame seeds
25 g (1 oz) sugar-free apricot jam

1. Boil the raisins in the water until the water is absorbed.

2. Mix the peanut butter, carob powder, sesame seeds, jam and raisins together.

3. Press into an 18 cm (7 inch) diameter round tin and chill for 2 hours.

4. Cut into slices and serve.

# Apple and Tofu Cheesecake G & W

## Makes 12 slices

1 quantity of seed pastry (see page 176)
*Filling*
450 g (1 lb) eating apples, chopped
200 g (7 oz) firm tofu
100 ml (4 fl oz) water
1 egg, whisked
2 tablespoons freshly squeezed lemon juice
1 teaspoon vanilla essence
1 teaspoon cinnamon
25 g (1 oz) ground almonds
25 g brown rice flakes

1.  Bake the pastry blind in a 23 cm (9 in) baking tin for 10 minutes at 180°C (350°F) gas mark 4.

2.  Combine the apple with the water and purée in a blender or food processor. Add the tofu and continue to blend until a thick paste is formed.

3.  Fold in the whisked egg, lemon juice, vanilla essence, cinnamon and ground almonds.

4.  Pour the mixture into the part-baked pastry case and sprinkle with brown rice flakes.

5.  Return to the oven at the same temperature for 30 minutes.

6.  Serve chilled.

# Banana Cake w

## Makes 16 slices

75 g (3 oz) dried dates
100 ml (4 fl oz) water
225 g (8 oz) banana, finely mashed
1 egg (size 3) whisked
75 g (3 oz) wholewheat flour (white if on a wholewheat-free
    diet)
25 g (1 oz) soya flour
50 g (2 oz) ground almonds
1 teaspoon bicarbonate of soda
½ teaspoon vanilla essence
150 ml (5 fl oz) low-fat natural yogurt

1.  Pre-heat the oven to 180°C (350°F) gas mark 4.

2.  Cook the dates in the water over a low heat until all the water
    has been absorbed. Blend in a food processor to a smooth
    paste.

3.  Mix the cooled paste with the banana and egg, then fold in the
    flours, ground almonds and bicarbonate of soda. Stir in the
    vanilla essence and yogurt.

4.  Lightly grease and flour a 20cm (8 inch) diameter baking tin
    and pour in the mixture.

5.  Bake for 35–40 minutes until the cake is brown on top and
    comes away from the tin.

# Pineapple Cake G & W

*Makes 12 slices*

50 g (2 oz) prunes, stoned and finely chopped
25 g (1 oz) dried figs
150 ml (5 fl oz) water
300 g (10 oz) fresh pineapple *or* tinned pineapple in fruit
    juice, drained
25 g (1 oz) raisins
40 g (1½ oz) pumpkin seeds
2 eggs, whisked well
40 g (1½ oz) ground almonds
75 g (3 oz) brown rice flour

1.  Pre-heat the oven to 180°C (350°F) gas mark 4.

2.  Place the prunes, figs and water in a saucepan and simmer
    until the water has been absorbed and the fruit is soft. Mash
    with a fork and leave to cool.

3.  Chop the pineapple into 1 cm (½ inch) squares, combine
    with the raisins and add the dried fruit paste.

4.  Grind the pumpkin seeds.

5.  Add the egg to the fruit mixture.

6.  Fold in the ground almonds, pumpkin seeds and flour.

7.  Pour the mixture into a greased and floured 20 cm (8 inch)
    baking tin.

8.  Bake for 40 minutes.

# Oatcakes W & Y

*Makes 12 square oatcakes*

50 g (2 oz) oatmeal
50 g (2 oz) oatgerm and bran
1 tablespoon vegetable oil
30 ml (2 tablespoons) concentrated apple juice
20 ml (2 dessert spoons) boiling water

1. Pre-heat the oven to 170°C (325°F) gas mark 3.

2. Combine the oatmeal, oatgerm, bran and oil in a bowl.

3. Add the apple juice and hot water to make a soft doughy mixture.

4. Roll out on a work top lightly dusted with oatmeal.

5. Cut into squares and place on an ungreased baking sheet.

6. Bake for 20 to 25 minutes.

# Seed Pastry G & W

1 tablespoon boiling water
50 g (2 oz) dried figs, chopped
25 g (1 oz) sunflower seeds
25 g (1 oz) pumpkin seeds
25 g (1 oz) sesame seeds, toasted
25 g (1 oz) ground hazelnuts
½ teaspoon mixed spice

1. Leave the figs to stand in the boiling water for 10 minutes.

2. Purée the figs in a blender or food processor.

3.  Grind all the seeds to powder and combine in a mixing bowl with the ground hazelnuts and mixed spices.

4.  Bind the seed mixture with the figs to make a dough. Add a little chilled water to bind if necessary.

5.  Roll out and prepare as ordinary pastry. This is an excellent sweet, grain-free pastry.

# Miss P's Punch G W & Y

*Makes 1 litre (1¾ pints)*

750 ml (1¼ pints) water
200 ml (⅓ pint) orange juice
50 ml (3–4 tablespoons) Ribena Light
2 yellow plums, chopped
2 red plums, chopped
1 orange, peeled, segmented and chopped
1 lemon, peeled and chopped
1 kiwi fruit, peeled and chopped
zest of 1 orange, peeled off in strips with a potato peeler or sharp knife.

Mix all the ingredients together and serve chilled. This makes a refreshing drink with or between meals, especially if served with ice on a hot day.

# RECOMMENDED READING LIST

## GENERAL HEALTH

1. *The Vitality Diet* by Dr Alan and Maryon Stewart, price £4.95 (published by Thorsons). **UK A**
2. *The Food Scandal* by Caroline Walker and Geoffrey Cannon, price £3.95 (published by Century Publishing Co). **UK A**
3. *Escape from Tranquillisers and Sleeping Pills* by Larry Neild, price £4.99 (published by Ebury Press). **UK**
4. *Pure, White and Deadly* by Professor John Yudkin (a book about sugar), price £9.95 (published by Viking). **UK A**
5. *Coming off Tranquillizers* by Dr Susan Trickett, price £1.99 (published by Thorsons). **UK USA A** (Lothian Publishing Co)
6. *The Better Pregnancy Diet* by Liz and Patrick Holford, price £3.95 (published by Ebury Press). **UK**
7. *The Migraine Revolution – The Drug-Free Solution* by Dr John Mansfield, price £3.99 (published by Thorsons). **UK USA A** (Lothian Publishing Co)
8. *The Book of Massage*, price £6.95 (published by Ebury Press). **UK**
9. *Do-it-yourself Shiatsu* by W. Ohashi, price £5.50 (published by Unwin). **UK**
10. *Shopping for Health* by Janette Marshall, price £3.95 (published by Pan Books). **UK**
11. *Nutritional Medicine* by Dr Stephen Davies and Dr Alan Stewart, price £6.99 (published by Pan Books). **UK A**
12. *Diet 2000* by Dr Alan Maryon-Davis with Jane Thomas, price £1.75 (published by Pan Books). **UK USA A**
13. *The Nutrition Detective* by Nan Kathryn Fuchs, price $16.95 (published by Jeremy P Tarcher, Inc). **USA**

14.  *Coping with Periods* by Dr Diana Sanders, price £2.95 (published by Chambers). **UK**
15.  *Pain-free Periods* by Stella Weller, price £2.50 (published by Thorsons). **UK**
16.  *Beat the Iron Crisis* by Leonard Mervyn, price £1.99 (published by Thorsons). **UK**
17.  *Brittle Bones and the Calcium Crisis* by Kathleen Mayes, price £4.99 (published by Thorsons). **UK**
18.  *Conquering Cystitis* by Dr Patrick Kingsley, price £3.95 (published by Ebury Press). **UK**
19.  *Alternative Health Care for Women* by Patsy Westcott, price £5.99 (published by Thorsons). **UK**
20.  *Food Irradiation: The Facts* by Tony Webb and Dr Tim Lang, price £1.99 (published by Thorsons). **UK**
21.  Parents For Safe Food *Safe Food Handbook* edited by Joan and Derek Taylor, price £6.99 (published by Ebury Press). **UK**

# DIET

1.  *The Food Allergy and Intolerance Diet* by Elizabeth Workman SRD, Dr John Hunter and Dr Virginia Alun Jones, price £3.95 (published by Optima Macdonald). **UK USA**
2.  *Food Combining for Health* by Doris Grant and Jean Joice, price £5.95 (published by Thorsons). **UK USA A** (Lothian Publishing Co)
3.  *Raw Energy* by Leslie and Susannah Kenton, price £2.25 (published by Century Publishing Co). **UK A** (Doubleday Publishing Co)
4.  *Foresight Index Number Decoder* (Packet Food Additive Dictionary), price £1.20, available from Foresight (address in Useful Address List page 182). **UK**
5.  *The Real Food and Restaurant Guide* by Clive Johnstone, price £3.95 (published by Ebury Press). **UK**
6.  *The Reluctant Vegetarian Cook* by Rose Elliot, price £8.95 (published by William Heinemann). **UK**
7.  *The Salt Free Diet Book* by Dr Graham MacGregor, price £3.95 (published by Martin Dunitz). **UK USA**
8.  *Gourmet Vegetarian Cooking* by Carole Handslip, price £2.95 (published by Fontana). **UK A**
9.  *Why You Don't Need Meat* by Peter Cox, price £2.50 (published by Thorsons). **UK A**

10. *Quantum Carrot, A New Concept in Small Space Organic Gardening* by Branton Kenton, price £5.95 (published by Ebury Press). **UK A**
11. *The Single Vegan* by Leah Leneman, price £4.99 (published by Thorsons). **UK**
12. *Bumper Bake Book* by Rita Greer, price £3.95 (published by Bunterbird Ltd, available from 225 Putney Bridge Road, London SW15 2PY). **UK**
13. *The New Organic Food Guide* by Alan Gear, price £3.95 (published by Dent Paperbacks). **UK A**
14. *The Arthritis Diet Cook Book* by Michael McIlwraith, price £4.95 (published by Gollancz). **UK**
15. *Organic Consumer Guide/Food you can trust*, Edited by David Mabey and Alan and Jackie Gear, price £4.99 (published by Thorsons). **UK USA A**

## STRESS

1. *Self Help for Your Nerves* by Dr Clair Weekes, price £5.95 (published by Angus and Robertson). **UK USA** (Hawthorn Publishing Co) **A**
2. *Stress Wise* by Dr Terry Looker and Dr Olga Gregson, price £4.95 (published by Headway, Hodder and Stoughton). **UK**

# USEFUL ADDRESSES

## GENERAL HEALTH

**Action Against Allergy**
23–24 George Street
Richmond
Surrey
TW9 1JY
(Postal enquiries, S.A.E.)

**Action on Phobias**
c/o Shandy Mathias
8–9 The Avenue
Eastbourne
Sussex
BN21 2YA
(Postal enquiries, S.A.E.)

**ASH (Action on Smoking and Health)**
5–11 Mortimer Street
London
W1N 7RH
Tel: London (071) 637 9843

**Alcoholics Anonymous (AA)**
General Services Office
PO Box 1
Stonebow House
Stonebow
York
YO1 2NJ
Tel: Stonebow (0904) 644026

**Anorexia and Bulimia Nervosa Association**
Tottenham Woman's and Health Centre
Annexe C, Tottenham Town Hall
London
N13 4RX
Tel: London (081) 885 3936
(Wednesdays 6–9 pm only)

**ASSET**
The National Association for Health and Exercise Teachers
202 The Avenue, Kennington
Oxford
OX1 5RN
Tel: Kennington (0865) 736066

**CLEAR (Campaign for Lead Free Air)**
3 Endsleigh Street
London
WC1H 0DD
Tel: London (071) 278 9686

**College of Health**
14 Buckingham Street
London
WC2N 6DS
Tel: London (071) 839 2413

**Foresight**
Association for the Promotion of
   Pre-Conceptual Care
The Old Vicarage
Church Lane
Whitney
Godalming
Surrey
GU8 5PM
Tel: Wormley (042879) 4500

**Food Watch International**
Butts Pond Industrial Estate
Sturminster Newton
Dorset
DT10 1AZ
Tel: Sturminster Newton (0258)
   73356

**Friends of the Earth Ltd**
26–28 Underwood Street
London
N1 8JQ
Tel: London (071) 490 1555

**Hyperactive Children Support
Group**
59 Meadowside
Angmering
Littlehampton
West Sussex
BN16 4BW
(Postal enquiries only)

**Julia Swift Exercise Studios**
Old Slipper Baths
North Road
Brighton
Sussex
Tel: Brighton (0273) 690016

**Migraine Trust**
45 Great Ormond Street
London
WC1 3HD
Tel: London (071) 278 2676

**Parents for Safe Food**
Britannia House
1/11 Glenthorne Road
London W6
Tel: London (081) 748 9898

**Samaritans**
17 Uxbridge Road
Slough
SL1 1SN
Tel: Slough (0753) 327133

**The Soil Association**
86–88 Colston Street
Bristol
BS1 5BB
Tel: Bristol (0272) 290661

**The Shiatsu Society**
Elaine Liechti
19 Langside Park, Kilbarchan
Renfrewshire
PA10 2EP
Tel: Kilbarchan (05057) 4657

**Tranx (UK) Ltd**
National Tranquilliser Advice
   Centre
Registered Office
25a Masons Avenue, Wealdstone
Harrow
Middlesex
HA3 5AH
Tel: client line (081) 427 2065
24 hour answering service (081)
427 2827

# WOMEN'S HEALTH

**Anorexic Support**
Norah Robinson-Smith
15 Sharnford Road
Leicestershire
Tel: Sapcote (045) 527 2398

**Association for Post-Natal Illness**
Gowan Avenue
London
SW6 6RH
Tel: London (071) 731 4867

**Birthright**
27 Sussex Place
London
NW1 4SP
Tel: London (071) 723 9296

**Brook Advisory Centres**
233 Tottenham Court Road
London
W1P 9AE
Tel: London (071) 580 2911/
    323 1522

**Caesarian Support Group**
Mrs D K Barnes
81 Elizabeth Way
Cambridge
CB4 1BQ
Tel: Cambridge (0223) 314211

**Endometriosis Society**
65 Holmdene Avenue
London
SE14 9LD
Tel: London (071) 737 4764

**Hysterectomy Support Group**
11 Henryson Road
Brockley
London
SE4 1HL
Tel: London (081) 690 5987

**Miscarriage Association**
Mrs K Ladley
18 Stoneybrook Close
West Bretton
Wakefield
West Yorkshire
WF4 4TP
Tel: Wakefield (092) 458 515

**National Osteoporosis Society**
Barton Meade House
PO Box 10
Radstock
Bath
BA3 3YB
Tel: Bath (0761) 32472

**Natural Family Planning Service**
Catholic Marriage Advisory Council
15 Lansdowne Road
London
W11 3AJ
Tel: London (071) 727 0141

**National Childbirth Trust**
Alexander House
Oldham
London
W3 6NH
Tel: London (081) 992 8637

**Pelvic Inflammatory Disease Group**
Ms P Fraser
c/o WRRIC, 52 Featherstone Street
London
EC1Y 8RT
Tel: London (071) 251 6333

**Pregnancy Advisory Service**
11–13 Charlotte Street
London
W1P 1HD
Tel: London (071) 637 8962

**Women's Health Information Centre**
52 Featherstone Street
London
EC1
Tel: London (071) 251 6580

**The Women's Nutritional Advisory Service**
PO Box 268
Hove, East Sussex
BN3 1RW
Tel: Hove (0273) 771366

# ALTERNATIVE HEALTH

**Aromatherapy – Guild of Practitioners**
123 Coombe Lane
London
SW20 0QY
Tel: London (081) 946 4643

**British Homeopathic Association**
27a Devonshire Street
London
W1N 1RJ
Tel: London (071) 935 2163

**British Acupuncture Register and Directory**
34 Alderney Street
London
SW1V 4EU
Tel: London (071) 834 1012

**British School of Osteopathy**
Little John House, 1–4 Suffolk Street
London
SW1 4HQ
Tel: London (071) 930 9234/8

**College of Health**
18 Victoria Park Square
London
E2 9PF
Tel: London (081) 980 6263

**Institute for Complementary Medicine**
21 Portland Place
London
W1N 3AF
Tel: London (071) 289 6111

**The European School of Osteopathy**
104 Tonbridge Road
Maidstone
Kent
ME16 8SL
Tel: Maidstone (0622) 671558

# NUTRITIONAL SUPPLEMENT SUPPLIERS

| UK | Supplies |
|---|---|
| *Name* | |
| **Efamol Nutrition**<br>Freepost, Efamol House, Woodbridge<br>Meadows, Guildford, Surrey GU21 1BR<br>Tel: Guildford (0483) 570860 | Efamol. |
| **Larkhall Laboratories Limited**<br>225–229 Putney Bridge Road,<br>London SW15 2PY<br>Tel: London (081) 874 1130 | A wide range of vitamins,<br>minerals and specialized<br>foods including Trufree flour. |
| **Health Crafts Limited**<br>45 Station Approach, West Byfleet,<br>Surrey KT14 6NE<br>Tel: West Byfleet (09323) 41133 | A wide range of vitamins<br>and minerals and specialized<br>foods. |
| **Nature's Best Health Products Ltd**<br>PO Box 1, Tunbridge Wells, Kent<br>TN2 3EQ<br>Tel: Tunbridge Wells (0892) 34143 | A wide range of vitamins<br>and minerals. Also Optivite. |
| **Nature's Own**<br>203–205 West Malvern Road, West<br>Malvern, Worcs WR14 4BB.<br>Tel: Malvern (0684) 892555 | A wide range of vitamins<br>and minerals. |

**Boots the Chemist**
All branches.

Optivite Magnesium
Hydroxide Mixture,
Efamol.

Practitioners can buy Chromium GTF from Lamberts.

*Australia*
**NNFA (National Nutrition Foods Association)**
PO Box 84, Westmead, NSW 2145. (tel: 02 633 9913).
The NNFA have lists of all supplement stockists and retailers in Australia, if you have any difficulties in obtaining supplements.
PMT Formula is available from **Blackmores**, 23 Roseberry Street, Balgowlah, NSW 2093, Australia (tel: 02 949 3177).

*New Zealand*
**NNFA (National Nutrition Foods Association)**
c/o PO Box 820062, Auckland, New Zealand.
Again the NNFA have lists of all supplement stockists and retailers in New Zealand, if you have any difficulties in obtaining supplements.
PMT Formula is available from **Blackmores**, 2 Parkhead Place, Albany, Auckland, (tel: 09 415 8585).

# INDEX